THE PMS DI

KAREN EVENNETT has been a freelance journalist for over ten years and specializes in writing about health and relationships for women's magazines. *The PMS Diet Book* is Karen's fourth book. She is the author of two other Sheldon titles, *Coping Successfully with PMS* and *Coping Successfully with Your Cervical Smear*, and *Women's Health: An Essential Guide for the Modern Woman*, published by Cassell. Karen loves good food, and her husband, Steve, a chef, has worked in some of London's top restaurants. They have two daughters, Coco and Bella, and live in Surrey.

Overcoming Common Problems Series

For a full list of titles please contact
Sheldon Press, Marylebone Road, London NW1 4DU

The Assertiveness Workbook
A plan for busy women
JOANNA GUTMANN

Birth Over Thirty Five
SHEILA KITZINGER

Body Language
How to read others' thoughts by their
gestures
ALLAN PEASE

Body Language in Relationships
DAVID COHEN

Cancer – A Family Affair
NEVILLE SHONE

Coping Successfully with Hayfever
DR ROBERT YOUNGSON

Coping Successfully with Migraine
SUE DYSON

Coping Successfully with Pain
NEVILLE SHONE

**Coping Successfully with Your Irritable
Bowel**
ROSEMARY NICOL

Coping with Anxiety and Depression
SHIRLEY TRICKETT

Coping with Breast Cancer
DR EADIE HEYDERMAN

Coping with Bronchitis and Emphysema
DR TOM SMITH

Coping with Chronic Fatigue
TRUDIE CHALDER

Coping with Depression and Elation
DR PATRICK McKEON

Curing Arthritis Diet Book
MARGARET HILLS

Curing Arthritis – The Drug-Free Way
MARGARET HILLS

Depression
DR PAUL HAUCK

Divorce and Separation
Every woman's guide to a new life
ANGELA WILLANS

**Everything Parents Should Know About
Drugs**
SARAH LAWSON

Good Stress Guide, The
MARY HARTLEY

Heart Attacks – Prevent and Survive
DR TOM SMITH

Helping Children Cope with Grief
ROSEMARY WELLS

How to Improve Your Confidence
DR KENNETH HAMBLY

How to Interview and Be Interviewed
MICHELE BROWN AND GYLES
BRANDRETH

How to Keep Your Cholesterol in Check
DR ROBERT POVEY

How to Pass Your Driving Test
DONALD RIDLAND

**How to Start a Conversation and Make
Friends**
DON GABOR

How to Write a Successful CV
JOANNA GUTMANN

Hysterectomy
SUZIE HAYMAN

The Irritable Bowel Diet Book
ROSEMARY NICOL

Overcoming Guilt
DR WINDY DRYDEN

The Parkinson's Disease Handbook
DR RICHARD GODWIN-AUSTEN

Talking About Anorexia
How to cope with life without starving
MAROUSHKA MONRO

Think Your Way to Happiness
DR WINDY DRYDEN AND JACK
GORDON

Overcoming Common Problems

THE PMS
DIET BOOK

Karen Evennett

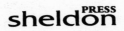

First published in Great Britain in 1997 by
Sheldon Press, SPCK, Marylebone Road, London NW1 4DU

British Library Cataloguing-in-Publication Data
A catalogue record for this book is available from the British
Library.

ISBN 0–85969–759–2

Photoset by Deltatype Limited, Birkenhead, Merseyside
Printed in Great Britain by
Biddles

Contents

Acknowledgements

My special thanks go to Gaynor Bussell and Dr Michael Brush, who both took time to read my manuscript and advise me on it. Their very kind words in the Foreword and cover copy are extremely encouraging, and I hope readers will be as inspired as they were by the recipes in this book.

Foreword

Premenstrual Syndrome, or PMS, can have a destructive effect on an individual, her family and society. It has a high prevalence rate: around 95 per cent of women of reproductive age suffer from it to some degree, 5 per cent of them to such an extent that their lives are totally disrupted for two weeks out of four. Today's woman may have as many as 500 menstrual cycles in her life. In view of these facts, a therapy for PMS which is safe, efficient and acceptable needs to be sought. For many, especially those whose diet is poor, good nutrition fulfils these criteria. In addition it allows the sufferer to participate in her own treatment and is a relatively cheap form of therapy.

At the least, dietary changes like those outlined in this book will improve a woman's general health and self-esteem, and may increase her tolerance of premenstrual changes and thus reduce the impact of PMS. If other methods are used to treat PMS, they are more likely to be successful if the diet is optimum. Furthermore, if a woman adopts a healthy-eating approach, it has a 'knock on' benefit for any who depend on her as the meal provider.

Not everyone will react in the same way to the dietary changes; for some fortunate women, small changes such as cutting down on fats will be all that is needed to bring relief. Other women may need to try some supplements before any benefits are perceived. Everyone is different.

At the PMS Clinic of the University College London Hospital I use a three-phase dietary approach which very much follows the healthy-eating guidelines of this book. To begin with, the sufferer is advised to cut down on fats, refined sugars, salt, alcohol and caffeinated beverages and to increase her consumption of starches and fibre.

It takes about three months for the diet to have a significant effect. If, after this time, there has been little or no improvement, phase two is introduced. This involves excluding refined sugars and starches as much as possible and trying to leave no more than three or four hours between meals. Each meal or snack should include something starchy. Although there is little evidence that true hypoglycaemia (abnormally low blood sugar levels) occurs in PMS subjects, many do experience 'hypo-type' symptoms, such as irritability, faintness, shakiness, severe hunger, sugar cravings and anxiety. Experience has shown that these symptoms can be relieved by regular carbohydrate consumption.

If after a month there is still no significant improvement, phase three is brought into play. This entails a vitamin and mineral cocktail tailored to the individual.

Underlying medical problems, such as allergies and food intolerances, diabetes, anaemia and irritable bowel, should also be appropriately treated through diet. Controlling such conditions will help to alleviate PMS.

The above dietary guidelines are based on scientific evidence. It is also reassuring to note that they exactly fit the Department of Health's guidelines for the Health of the Nation, published in 1992. The only drawback to the dietary approach is that it may take time and patience before results are seen, but, as any sufferer will agree, it is certainly worth persevering in order to gain relief from the misery of PMS.

Gaynor Bussell, B.Sc. Hons., State Registered Dietician, Women's Health Dietician and Co-ordinator of the National Association for Premenstrual Syndrome's Dietary Advisory Team

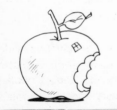

PART ONE

1

Is it PMS?

If you think you suffer from PMS, the first thing you need to know is that you are not alone. Premenstrual Syndrome is the most common illness to affect women of childbearing age: nine out of ten of us suffer from it, to some degree, at some point in our lives.

However, accepting that, as a sufferer, you are in the majority of women will be of little consolation unless you are prepared to use this information to your advantage and work with your body and symptoms towards finding a suitable treatment. Whether this involves self-help, over-the-counter remedies, or medical intervention, you are bound to discover along the way that a change of diet will also be of enormous value.

The aims of this book are to describe the benefits of a healthy anti-PMS diet and to show that the dietary changes involved need not be complicated – or unpalatable.

Before launching yourself into a new regime, you will need to understand what PMS is and how it manifests itself. In this chapter I answer some of the questions which are discussed in more detail in my earlier book, *Coping Successfully with PMS*.

Understanding your menstrual cycle

Although the exact cause of PMS has not been identified, we do know that it is linked to the hormonal changes which take place during the menstrual cycle. In a normal healthy and fertile woman, the menstrual cycle usually lasts around 28 days, although slightly shorter or longer cycles are still acceptable and entirely 'normal' (the official gynaecological definition of the length of the menstrual cycle is 21–35 days).

The cycle follows the same pattern every month (unless pregnancy takes place) as an ovum (egg) develops and is released from a small sac or cyst, called a follicle, within one of the ovaries. The release of the ovum is called ovulation and happens during the

3

middle of the menstrual cycle, usually between days 10 and 14 of a typical 28-day cycle.

The egg grows inside the follicle. By the time it is ready to be released, this follicle will have reached about 2.5 cm (1 inch) in diameter. If you were examined on an ultrasound scan immediately before ovulation, the follicle would show on the ovary. This is entirely normal.

When the follicle ruptures, the fluid inside it leaks into the abdominal cavity. Some blood may also escape from the follicle and this too will normally spill into the abdomen and be disposed of through the body's natural waste system.

The egg then begins its journey through the Fallopian tube to the uterus. If it is not fertilized, the egg dies and, along with its accompanying mucus and blood, is disposed of during the next period, at which point the cycle starts all over again.

Throughout the monthly cycle, there is an enormous amount of hormonal activity in your body as it undergoes an amazing number of changes. The coordination of these changes is timed with the precision of a busy airport runway and controlled by the hypothalamus, a small cherry-shaped structure at the base of the brain. The hypothalamus is responsible for sending chemical messengers (hormones) all over the body. It controls the secretion of hormones from the pituitary gland, to which it is connected by a short stalk of nerve fibres.

The menstrual cycle starts when the hypothalamus sends a message to the pituitary gland giving it the go-ahead to produce its own hormones. The first of these, follicle stimulating hormone (FSH), is carried in the bloodstream to the ovaries. Once there, it stimulates the growth of the follicle within which the egg develops.

As the egg grows, the walls of the follicle produce increasing amounts of the female hormone oestrogen. This starts to thicken the lining of the uterus (womb), and often causes increased sexual interest as the level of oestrogen in the blood builds up to a peak just before ovulation.

The pituitary gland now releases another hormone, luteinizing hormone (LH), which triggers ovulation – the release of the mature egg. As the egg begins to travel from the ovary through the Fallopian tube to the uterus, the LH turns the follicle into a solid mass of yellow tissue known as the corpus luteum, which produces large amounts of progesterone. The main function of this hormone is to prepare the lining of the uterus to receive the fertilized egg.

If the egg is not fertilized, the pituitary gland, responding to the high level of oestrogen and progesterone produced by the corpus luteum in the ovary, will reduce its production of LH. The drop in LH causes the corpus luteum to decay, and the levels of progesterone and oestrogen then fall too.

What is happening to the cycle when PMS occurs?

The symptoms of PMS are experienced during the latter half of the menstrual cycle, after ovulation has taken place, when it is thought that there is either too much or too little of certain hormones in the woman's body.

Possible causes of PMS

Too little progesterone

One of the most popular theories about PMS has been that it is due to a deficiency of the hormone progesterone in relation to the amount of oestrogen in the body in the second half of the cycle.

A lot of women benefit greatly from treatment with progesterone therapy, which boosts natural supplies of progesterone at this crucial stage in the cycle. However, this treatment does not work for everyone, and some women with very severe symptoms of PMS have perfectly normal levels of progesterone.

Too much oestrogen

Excessively high levels of oestrogen have been thought to cause depression and mood swings. Oestrogen interferes with the body's utilization of vitamin B_6, which is known as the anti-depression vitamin because it controls the production of a compound called serotonin. Serotonin is essential for brain and nerve function and an inadequate supply causes depression.

Too much prolactin

Prolactin is the hormone produced by the pituitary gland to regulate levels of oestrogen and progesterone. It also stimulates the breasts to produce milk when you have had a baby. An excess of prolactin, which is very unusual, can make your breasts sore and enlarged, and can also upset the delicate balance of progesterone and oestrogen.

Too few essential fatty acids

Studies have shown that where essential fatty acids (EFAs) are in short supply, the body is abnormally sensitive to small changes in hormonal levels, leading to the same symptoms as those produced by an excess of prolactin.

A deficiency of vitamin B_6

A hormone imbalance can affect the way your body uses its supplies of vitamin B_6. Vitamin B_6, in turn, increases the efficiency with which your body makes use of EFAs. If you have a hormone imbalance, you may need more than the usual amount of vitamin B_6 in your diet.

A problem with the hypothalamus

The best way to describe the hypothalamus connection is to repeat an analogy I used in *Coping Successfully with PMS*. Imagine the hormones are the planes taking off and landing at a busy airport, and that each of these is in perfect working order, with an A1 pilot in the cockpit. If, nevertheless, a crash does occur, you would probably start your investigation back in the air traffic control centre.

Like the air traffic control centre, the hypothalamus is responsible for receiving and sending out messages. It has only to get one or two lines crossed during the menstrual cycle and your normal hormonal activity will be sent off course, causing PMS.

A problem with the pituitary gland

It is possible that an underactive pituitary gland, one step further along the line, is at the root of some women's PMS. A poor diet can cause the activity of this gland to decrease and, in severe cases, periods may stop altogether. Physical or emotional stress can also cause the pituitary gland to put its feet up and stop working as hard as it should.

Why do some women suffer from PMS while others do not?

Symptoms of PMS may be mild and hardly noticeable, but sometimes they are so severe that they take over the sufferer's whole life, and their cause is not recognized. What seems particularly unfair is that while some women suffer in the extreme from PMS, others go through life without any symptoms.

Just as, within a family, one person can be taller or shorter than their brothers and sisters, and another's freckles or hairy legs make them the odd one out, a woman's internal systems can work differently to those of her sisters, mother and grandmothers.

It seems that some of us are simply more vulnerable than others to the many factors, including diet, lifestyle and pollution, that seem to play some part in blocking or increasing the production of the key hormones which control the menstrual cycle and premenstrual changes within that cycle.

Even if all the female members of one family suffer from PMS, each woman's symptoms may stem from a different cause, or originate from a different point on the menstrual circuit. And it is because there are so many possible causes for PMS that finding the most suitable treatment can be a long-drawn-out process.

Recognizing the warning signs

Psychologists have identified a total of 150 symptoms which may appear alone or in batches in the days (or, in some cases, weeks) leading up to a woman's period. Many of these overlap with each other or are very rare. The most common symptoms are:

- feeling depressed, sad, or pessimistic
- feeling under par, tired or lethargic
- tension, irritability and anxiety
- a change in appetite
- cravings for sugary or salty foods
- poor concentration
- mood swings
- indecisiveness
- weepiness
- feeling extra sexy or losing interest in sex
- sleeping badly
- aggression
- impulsiveness
- increased energy in the days leading up to a period
- loss of confidence and self-esteem
- feelings of guilt and inadequacy
- headaches and/or migraine
- swollen, tender breasts
- bloating
- swollen fingers and toes
- constipation, nausea or diarrhoea
- clumsiness
- muscle weakness and backache
- dizziness
- weight gain
- a change in the amount of urine passed
- abdominal cramps
- feeling less efficient than usual.

What type of PMS sufferer are you?

In the 1980s, Professor Guy Abrahams, formerly Professor of Obstetrics and Gynaecology at the University of California, and now patron of the Women's Nutritional Advisory Service, identified four types of PMS sufferer:

Type A experience anxiety, irritability and tension.
Type B experience bloating, swelling and weight gain.

Type C experience cravings for sweets and stodgy foods followed by exhaustion, headache and fainting brought on by hypoglycaemia (sudden rises and falls in blood sugar).

Type D experience depression and confusion.

Most sufferers experience symptoms from more than one of these groups.

Nervous tension, anxiety, irritability and mood swings are thought to be caused by elevated levels of oestrogen in the premenstrual phase, due to a vitamin B_6 deficiency. The liver, which breaks down the body's waste products, needs healthy supplies of vitamin B_6 in order to get rid of the portion of oestrogen which is no longer needed in the second half of the menstrual cycle. If, for some reason, you lack the necessary levels of vitamin B_6, the liver cannot do its job properly and oestrogen builds up in the body.

Too much oestrogen is thought to cause an imbalance in brain chemicals and over-production of the stimulating chemicals, such as serotonin, adrenalin and noradrenalin, and under-production of the soothing chemicals, such as dopamine. With these chemicals out of balance, you are likely to feel irritable and 'uptight' and to suffer dramatic mood swings: you may fluctuate between being bad-tempered and aggressive and feeling drowsy and incapable of performing everyday tasks at your normal capacity, for example.

Bloating, swelling and weight gain are caused by fluid retention, which is also a symptom of too much oestrogen. Even dieters may notice that their weight, which has been falling steadily, suddenly soars premenstrually. Scientists have observed that oestrogen causes the body to retain high levels of sodium, which is found in salt. The sodium causes water to remain in the body; instead of being excreted as usual it finds its way into other parts of the body, causing fingers to swell, breasts to balloon, waistlines to expand and ankles to thicken up. Swelling in the nose can make you feel stuffed-up, as if you have a cold. And a build-up of water in the sinuses may produce a headache.

Cravings and attacks of nausea and tiredness are common features of PMS and are symptoms of hypoglycaemic attacks. The question is, why should premenstrual women experience hypogly-caemic attacks more than anyone else?

What normally happens is that our blood sugar level rises quickly after eating and then falls gradually over a period of hours until the next meal, by which time our blood sugar level has reached its 'baseline' and we are usually feeling tired and in need of pepping up.

Premenstrually, it seems that changes in the hormone levels affect our normal sugar tolerance, causing the blood sugar baseline to rise so that we cannot manage to go without food as long as we normally would. One way of getting the quick burst of energy your body is telling you it needs is to eat something sweet. Hence a lot of women experience chocolate cravings at this time of the month.

Unfortunately, chocolate and sugary foods actually exacerbate the problem. They give you short bursts of excitable high energy, followed by a sudden fit of weakness, lethargy and hunger (as your blood sugar level suddenly drops back) which make us crave even more chocolate or sugar. Soon you are locked into a vicious circle of cravings and attacks of nausea.

Depression and confusion, insomnia and weepiness are caused not by the high levels of oestrogen linked to other symptoms of PMS, but by low levels during the first half of the menstrual cycle. One reason for these low levels is thought to be that lead poisoning, which has been linked to depression, blocks the production of oestrogen. Stress is also thought to affect the production of this hormone and many PMS sufferers report aggravated symptoms when they are under stress.

Triggers

Factors which can predispose you to PMS by causing problems with your fluctuating hormone levels include:

- stressful life events (illness, marital discord, overwork, etc.)
- childbirth
- postnatal depression

- recent gynaecological operations, a miscarriage or an abortion
- drinking alcohol
- smoking cigarettes
- pollution (because coping with it drains your natural supply of PMS-fighting nutrients)
- gynaecological disorders such as endometriosis or ovarian cysts
- a psychiatric disorder
- a tendency towards mental illness (because of heritable psychiatric disorders in the family, for example)
- lack of exercise
- a diet of processed (especially sugary) foods
- a high-fat diet
- long-term use of the Pill sometimes causes small deficiencies in your nutritional stocks which can go unnoticed, because the Pill stops ovulation, but which will give you sudden PMS when you finally come off the Pill
- your age – PMS symptoms are known to get worse as you get older
- a food allergy or sensitivity.

PMS diaries and charts

If you suspect your problems are associated with PMS, and are serious about getting the treatment you need, you may feel you have to prove your case to your GP. One way of doing this is to invest in a spacious diary and, over the course of three months, keep a daily note of:

- Your emotions. For example, 'irritable', 'weepy', 'depressed'. Even if you do not feel that your emotions are noteworthy, do record any upsets or arguments you have had and the subject of them. 'Cashier rude to me in Sainsbury's', or 'Furious with children for being late getting up for school' may later translate as a big fuss over nothing.
- Any physical symptoms, such as headache, nausea, bloating, sore breasts, fatigue, spottiness, mouth ulcers.

- What you ate. For example, 'Breakfast: coffee, toast, butter, jam. Lunch: cheese and tomato sandwich. Supper: spaghetti bolognese and salad.'
- What you drank. Try to keep a record of all fluids consumed. For example, 'Morning: three cups of coffee. Lunch: Coke. Afternoon: three cups of tea. Evening: two glasses of red wine.'
- Any exercise you took. For example, 'Walked the dog, cycled to the shops, swimming class in evening.' If you didn't leave the house, say so. Be honest with your diary – it's for your own good!
- Any current stress or worries in your life. For example, 'Worried about money today', 'A lot of work on; late leaving office.'

At the end of each week, on a separate monthly chart, make a note of the main physical and emotional symptoms you have suffered, and also the dates when your period started and finished.

Charting symptoms is an important key to diagnosis, since it provides an at-a-glance picture of when the symptoms occur during the menstrual cycle, which symptoms are linked to the cycle and which are present at other times too. Invariably women who keep a chart realize that some of the symptoms they thought were premenstrual actually occurred throughout the whole month, while symptoms they did not associate with PMS are in fact surprisingly relevant!

Don't look on keeping your diary and charts as a chore. Together, they will help you identify precisely when and how you are experiencing PMS. Your notes about diet and exercise may also give you clues about how best to alleviate some of your symptoms. You may notice, for example, that you are drinking a lot of coffee, which you could replace with water, fruit juice or herb teas, or that you are eating too little fibre and too much meat and dairy fat.

2

How can diet help?

In the last chapter I explained the importance of keeping a diary and charts to help identify symptoms which may be premenstrual. At the end of three months a pattern to your symptoms will have emerged. By transferring your notes from your diary to your chart, you will be able to pick out this pattern very clearly.

You may by this stage have already reached the conclusion that self-help will be better for you than medical intervention. Even if this is the case, I would recommend at least one trip to your GP, with your diaries and charts, so that any more serious condition can be ruled out.

Unless your symptoms are extremely severe, your doctor may also suggest self-help treatments as a first resort, such as vitamins, minerals and evening primrose oil. The more drastic 'remedies' include hormonal treatments, antiprostaglandins, diuretics, anti-depressants and tranquillizers.

However, because PMS is still so poorly understood by a great number of doctors, the medical treatments suggested may not always be those that a PMS expert would recommend. Further-more, as a general rule, you should remember that there is no single magic treatment which works for everyone. The process of finding the right treatment may be a long one. You may start off with vitamin supplements and end up with progesterone supposi-tories. Better this way round than to start with unnecessary medication. Better still, you may find that all you need is a change in diet.

Certainly, PMS seems to be a classic example of a twentieth-century disease, exacerbated by our modern diet and lifestyle. We consume far too much sugar, salt and animal fats, and our bodies are under extra stress from the pollutants we have to cope with, such as lead in petrol fumes or old lead plumbing, and pesticides in crop sprays.

What do these things have to do with our hormonal cycles?

Quite a lot, in fact. In Chapter 1 I explained how the hypothalamus and pituitary gland control the hormones which govern the menstrual cycle. As well as controlling hormone production, the hypothalamus regulates appetite, hunger and thirst. It also operates by feedback, that is, by responding to what is already happening in the body. The action of the hypothalamus is affected by trauma, nutrition and infection.

Nutritional deficiencies, whether due entirely to a poor diet, or depleted by external pollutants, have the capacity to disturb the whole system. Diet is important for another reason too. The hypothalamus responds to neurotransmitters, the substances which we secrete under stress and which are related to mood changes, and it is known that diet can directly affect the way we cope with stress.

In Chapter 4 I will discuss in detail the dietary changes you should be aiming for, but here are some general tips:

- Make sure your energy levels are constant by eating plenty of high-fibre foods, such as brown rice, wholemeal pasta, vegetables and baked potatoes.
- Cut down on sugary foods, which produce mood swings via fluctuating energy levels.
- Cut out caffeine, which speeds up adrenalin production, adding to the 'charging' or 'racing' feeling experienced with stress.
- Stop smoking. Smoking depletes the body's supplies of vitamin B_6.
- Don't drink alcohol, which contributes to mood swings and exacerbates insomnia, lethargy and depression.

Changing to a healthy new regime will be easy if you stick to four ground rules:

1. *Don't cut anything right out of your diet*
Variety is the key to an interesting diet. It should also provide you with all the nutrients you need. Rather than dropping things from your usual shopping list, try to swap them for new alternatives. You will probably also have to adjust the ratio of foods you eat.

14

Instead of using vegetables as a garnish to mainly meat and dairy meals, try to make them a substantial feature of your new menu. Plan your meals around the staples. For example, 'Tonight we'll have pasta/baked potatoes/rice.' Then add vegetables and a moderate amount of protein. Be adaptable. You can still use your favourite old recipes, but use yoghurt instead of cream, low-fat milk instead of whole milk, low-fat instead of full-fat cheese, and so on.

2. *Be adventurous*
Try out new foods and different cooking methods. Eastern cookery tends to be low in fat and high in fibre. Buy yourself some new cookery books and see what you can learn from other cultures.

3. *Be positive*
If you let your diet make you miserable, you will find it hard to make the necessary changes for a healthier regime. Remember, the reason you've changed your diet is to improve your life, not wreck it.

4. *Take one step at a time*
It is far easier to make the changes gradually. That way they will slowly become part of your life. Be gentle with yourself and don't expect an overnight transformation.

3

The bad PMS diet

I find it impossible to think about the bad PMS diet without recalling the birthday cake my husband once made for our daughter. It was rich, dark and chocolatey, and far too sophisticated for the children, who all turned up their noses at it and left huge chunks on their plates. Their parents, however, eagerly polished off the leftovers. When our guests were leaving, one of the mothers sheepishly asked, 'Could I have the recipe for that PMS cake?'

She, like many of the women I talked to when I was writing *Coping Successfully with PMS*, experienced severe chocolate cravings every month when she was premenstrual. The problem was, she had no idea her eating habits were exacerbating her PMS.

In my book, Joyce, one of my case histories, describes how one day she'd rushed into work, desperate to make herself a chocolate drink:

> . . . Joyce's relief was instant as she took her first, long, sip.
>
> She was still savouring the moment when the cleaning lady popped her head round the door.
>
> 'Hot chocolate, at this time of day?' she teased.
>
> 'Yes,' Joyce laughed. 'I could have murdered for it this morning!' Then she added, 'I bet you anything I'm exactly ten days off from my period.'
>
> Joyce recalls: 'The cleaning lady looked completely baffled as I rushed back to my desk and returned with my diary. "Told you so!" I said as we both stared at my chart. There, in black and white was my period, marked with a cross, exactly ten days ahead.'

Other women have described driving out at night, in the kind of weather the rest of us would avoid like the plague, to track down a late-night garage selling chocolate, or eating several big bars of chocolate in one sitting.

Chocolate isn't the only thing we crave premenstrually. Cola drinks, crisps, salted peanuts and even Cornish pasties have found their way into the premenstrual larder. While providing the temporary 'lift' we desire, these foods make our symptoms far worse.

Maintaining blood sugar levels

Many women who suffer from PMS have found that their symptoms are exacerbated by low blood sugar levels. Keeping blood sugar at a safe level is therefore essential if treatment of PMS is to be successful, but eating chocolates and sweet and salty snacks is not the way to do this.

The blood sugar level is the ratio of glucose to blood produced when carbohydrates (found in sugars, rice, potatoes, bread and cereals) are broken down in the digestive system. Glucose, the result of this breaking-down process, passes into the bloodstream. The pancreas then releases insulin to help keep the amount of sugar in the blood at normal levels.

It has been found that attacks of aggression, panic, migraine and so on are more likely to occur when there are long intervals between meals or when meals contain insufficient or no carbohydrate. This causes a fall in the blood sugar level, followed by the release of a spurt of adrenalin, which allows the blood sugar level to be topped up by some of the glucose from the body's stores. This process continues until more carbohydrate is eaten. In women suffering from PMS this release of adrenalin occurs more often.

Blood sugar is affected not only by the amount of carbohydrate eaten, but also by the type. If your diet consists mainly of refined carbohydrates (sugar, sweets and chocolates, cakes, white flour and polished rice), the breakdown to glucose is much quicker than if your diet is rich in unrefined carbohydrates (wholemeal bread, wholemeal flour, brown rice, high-fibre breakfast cereals such as shredded wheat and porridge, pulses, jacket potatoes, fruit and vegetables).

The most sensible diet is a high-fibre diet, rich in unrefined carbohydrates. These will give you a sustained rise in blood glucose with the consequent better regulation of your blood sugar levels. Fibre also lowers oestrogen levels by preventing their reabsorption into the bloodstream, and it also helps combat constipation (a common symptom of PMS).

Sweet and salty foods

Salt and sugar are our worst enemies when they are hidden away in processed foods. Read the nutritional information labels on packaged foods and try to avoid those that contain added sugar and salt.

Try to use less salt during cooking (and preferably sea salt, which is lower in sodium than table salt) and none at the table. If you find this difficult, try buying a salt-cellar with smaller holes: people tend to shake for the same amount of time, regardless of the amount of salt they're actually sprinkling on their food.

Steam vegetables instead of boiling them. Steaming enhances their flavour and you won't miss the salt you add when you boil them. Use herbs and spices in casseroles and other dishes as alternative flavourings.

Salty foods cause a further problem in women who suffer from premenstrual bloating. As I explained in Chapter 1, an excess of oestrogen causes water to remain in the body and find its way into fingers, ankles and waistline. The result is that you swell up and look and feel much heavier than usual. This is thought to be because high levels of oestrogen interfere with the body's production of aldosterone, a corticosteroid which, in excess, causes the body to retain salt and water. A low-salt diet can help considerably.

Cut down on sweet foods by making them part of a meal, and restrict them to once a day only. Dried fruit and 'sweet' spices, like cinnamon, nutmeg and cloves, can taste just as good in baking as sugar, and they're much better for you.

Caffeine

Caffeine is found in tea, coffee, cola drinks and chocolate as well as in some painkillers and cough and cold medicines. It acts as a stimulant and can cause anxiety, nervousness, irritability and depression. If you suffer from PMS, you may find that your symptoms are aggravated by caffeine. This is because the hormone oestrogen hinders the breakdown of caffeine. Heavy consumption of caffeine drinks combined with high levels of oestrogen (which are the root of the problem for many women) intensify the nervous symptoms of PMS.

The best way to cut down on caffeine is to limit the number of caffeine drinks (especially coffee, which seems to be more culpable than tea in triggering anxiety) you take in a day, especially after midday. Limiting yourself to one 'get-up-and-go' morning coffee is excellent. You will soon feel less nervous and stressed.

Cigarettes

Smoking should be avoided as it can deplete the body's vitamin B_6, which is needed to counteract many of the symptoms of PMS. But smoking is like every other addiction: once you are hooked it seems impossible to give up. You may have no desire to give up, in which case nothing in this book will convince you that you should. Or you may recognize that, while you are a committed smoker who cannot even contemplate a future without cigarettes, your friends and family may feel differently. They may want you to seek help and give up smoking.

You may even be ready to quit, having – for health, financial or social reasons – reached the conclusion that you must stop smoking. But, as you will have learned, reaching that decision is only half the battle. The question now is, how to go about quitting. Whichever way you choose, it won't be easy, but it will be worth it. And the good news is that in the U.K. alone there are over 11 million ex-smokers. If they can do it, so can you!

You have two habits to break. One is your addiction to nicotine. The other is your habit of lighting up. Alternative therapies such as hypnotherapy and acupuncture help some people to stop smoking. There are also products such as nicotine patches you can try.

Nicotine replacement treatments

These reduce some of the withdrawal symptoms you feel when you stop smoking cigarettes by giving you a low blood nicotine level. They include:

Nicotine gum

You can buy 2 mg nicotine gum from the chemist. Alternatively, stronger (4 mg) gum is available on private prescription from your doctor. Nicotine gum helps by curbing withdrawal symptoms and giving you something to do. But there is a risk of becoming addicted to the gum, and it can cause mild jaw ache, indigestion and nausea.

Nicotine patches

You can buy these patches in three strengths. They look like plasters and are stuck on your arm, chest or back, where they slowly release nicotine into the body through the skin. They are easy to use, and the fact that there is no instant 'buzz' means you are less likely to become addicted to the patches, although you may still get an uncontrollable urge to have a cigarette.

Nicotine lozenges and tablets

These are intended to be taken in place of a cigarette every time you get the desire to light up. They have not yet been proven to be particularly beneficial, but neither are they thought to be useless.

All nicotine replacement products carry side-effects, such as vivid dreams, disturbed sleep and nausea, but for some people they provide the perfect stopgap, helping to break their addiction.

Non-nicotine products

These include:

Herbal cigarettes

Although nicotine-free, these cigarettes still produce carbon monoxide and tar. They should be seen as a short-term alternative to cigarettes; you use them to replace cigarettes then gradually cut down the herbal cigarettes too. There are some fears that they could be harmful.

Filters
These remove some of the tar and nicotine from cigarette smoke.

Silver acetate products
These include chewing gums and mouthwashes designed to make smoking taste unpleasant.

Advice from QUIT

According to QUIT, the charity which is committed to offering practical help to people who want to stop smoking, the best way to give up is to stop smoking altogether, not to do so gradually.

Here are QUIT's ten steps to stopping smoking:

1. Make a date to stop smoking completely – and stick to it.
2. Keep yourself busy to help you get through the first few days. Throw away all your ashtrays, unopened cigarette packets, matches and lighters.
3. Drink lots of water, and keep a glass by your side from which you can sip steadily.
4. Be more active. This will help you relax. Join an exercise class, go for a walk or have a swim.
5. Think positive. Withdrawal signs, although unpleasant, should be welcomed because they are positive signs that your body is recovering from the effects of tobacco. Common symptoms include headaches, sore throats and irritability. They will all disappear within a week or two.
6. Change your routine. If you bought your cigarettes on your usual route to work, go another way for a few days. If you smoked with friends at the pub at lunchtime, go somewhere else and do something different.
7. Don't make excuses. A crisis or a celebration is no excuse for 'just one' cigarette. One leads to another, and another.
8. Treat yourself. Use the money you've saved by not buying cigarettes for something special.

9. Watch what you eat. Eat fruit instead of fatty snacks if you're feeling peckish.
10. Take one day at a time and remember, each day is good news for your health, your family and your pocket.

For extra support, call the QUITLINE on 0800 002200. They can put you in touch with someone to talk to on the phone or a local stop-smoking group made up of other people in the same boat, all of whom want to boost their chances of success.

Alcohol

Alcohol contains high levels of sugar so consuming it contributes to mood swings brought about by fluctuating blood sugar levels. It is also a depressant of the central nervous system and can exacerbate insomnia, which also causes lethargy, clumsiness and depression. On top of this it inhibits the body's production of gamma-linolenic acid (GLA).

Cutting down

- If you drink more than 14 units of alcohol a week, you might find it worth keeping a drink diary to monitor when, where and with whom you drink the most. This will help you work out ways of cutting down.
- Try to keep one or two days a week alcohol-free.
- Sip drinks slowly.
- Stick to smaller measures.
- Don't feel obliged to keep up with other drinkers.

If you're finding it hard to cut down, confidential advice and guidance are available from a number of organizations. (See the addresses at the end of this book.)

4

The good PMS diet

OK, so you've read about cutting down on chocolate, cakes, alcohol, cigarettes, coffee and salty snacks. By now, if you're like the many PMS sufferers I've spoken to in the past, you are probably gasping for a fix. How will you cope without your lifelines?

In *Coping Successfully with PMS*, Carole describes how she dealt with this question. She had written to the Women's Nutritional Advisory Service (WNAS) asking how she could cure her premenstrual mood swings.

As well as some special foods to which the WNAS thought Carole might be sensitive, she was asked to give up caffeine, chocolate, cakes, cigarettes and alcohol. This is how she reacted.

I dropped all these baddies overnight, which was perhaps a bit rash, as I experienced awful withdrawal symptoms for a week. Then I began to think, 'Is this really worth it?'

One morning at the end of that first week, I woke up feeling so rotten that I just got up, made the breakfast, then crawled back to bed – where I stayed all day and all night. But when I got up the following day, I felt fantastic! I hadn't felt that good in ages!

As with any diet, the first few months were the hardest. But the longer I was on it, the better I felt. Now, I have gradually reintroduced foods into my diet and can eat more or less anything I like – in moderation. I can actually control the way I feel with the things I eat.

When I look back, I can't believe how awful I used to feel. Today, I feel wonderful. I am confident, lively and energetic. And, best of all, those mood swings have gone . . . for good!

What is a good PMS diet?

Cutting unwholesome foods out of your diet is only worth while if you replace them with healthy foods, eaten in small, regular, meals. Remember, eating every three hours is an important key to preventing premenstrual mood swings. Try to take the time and effort to maintain this habit; you may, for example, need to take in a snack you can eat at your desk at work. Regular meals and snacks will help build up your resistance to PMS and stop you from craving the baddies which used to disturb your hormonal system.

For a generally healthy diet you should aim to eat:

- fresh rather than preserved, packaged or convenience foods
- plenty of vegetables and fruit (at least five helpings a day), preferably raw or lightly cooked to preserve nutritious value
- whole-grain products instead of refined foods, such as whole-grain bread and brown rice instead of white bread and white (polished) rice
- less red meat and more white meat, fish and pulses
- no more than 35 per cent of total calories from fats – polyunsaturated fats and vegetable oils rather than saturated fats
- as little sugar and salt as possible
- plenty of potatoes in their skins, pasta and brown rice to fill you up.

In addition to these commonsense rules, Dr Michael Brush, Chairman of The Premenstrual Society, recommends the following dietary guidelines for fighting PMS:

- All foods should be non-toxic for our bodies, that is, they should not contain artificial flavours, colours, preservatives or other food additives used cosmetically to enhance the appearance of food and increase sales. Make a habit of reading the food labels when shopping and reject any that contain additives.
- A high salt intake aggravates PMS, especially the bloating aspect of it. Resisting the craving for salty foods can reduce the severity of your symptoms.
- Giving in to a craving for sweets and sugary foods can result in

hypoglycaemia-like attacks after the brief 'lift' given by the sugar. The symptoms of low blood sugar can accentuate the PMS symptoms of depression, agitation, fatigue, irritability and headaches that are exactly like hypoglycaemic episodes.

- Prevent sweet cravings by eating small and regular amounts of natural carbohydrates (fresh fruit, pulses, whole grains, etc.). The body was not designed to handle refined sugar in concentrated forms such as chocolates and cakes.
- A diet which provides more protein than the body needs can cause severe deficiencies in many essential vitamins, including vitamin B_6 and niacin. Too much protein actually drains important minerals such as calcium, iron, zinc, phosphorus and magnesium from the body. Sixty grams ($2\frac{1}{2}$ oz) of protein a day should be sufficient.
- Aim to include in your diet foods rich in essential fatty acids, such as seeds and nuts, grains and fish (especially oily fish like mackerel). Avoid eating too many animal fats (saturated fats), which are found in butter, ordinary margarine, cheese and fatty meat.

You will not see the benefits of a change in diet overnight – it takes two to four months to get lasting results – but if you stray from the path of the good diet, you may pay the penalty within a few weeks.

Putting the good PMS diet into practice

Make the most of your microwave

Over a half of British households own a microwave oven. In many of these homes the microwave's sole job is to heat up pre-prepared meals in minutes, but it can be used to cook fresh and healthy meals just as quickly. With a microwave:

- baked potatoes can be ready in minutes,
- fish is tasty, firm and needs no added oil or fat, and
- fresh vegetables retain nutrients which are easily lost if boiled.

Make it a high-fibre diet

Of all the diet books to hit the best-seller lists, Audrey Eyton's *F-Plan Diet*, published in 1982, has had the greatest and most beneficial effect on the way we eat today. For years dieters had been looking for a miracle substance that would help them to lose weight, and Audrey Eyton's F-plan showed them that the very thing they wanted had been right under their noses all along: the natural fibre in food.

In fact, despite all the hype her diet received, the F-plan was anything but 'faddy'. Everything she said made complete sense. People in the developing world had a lower incidence of heart disease, digestive illness and obesity than those in the affluent West. One reason is that their diets were rich in the natural fibre ours lacked.

By the early eighties most of us were locked into a pattern of buying and eating mostly processed foods from which the fibre had been removed: white bread, cornflakes and white rice, for example. Our average intake of fibre was just 20 grams (less than 1 oz) a day, compared to a typical 50–120 grams (2–5 oz) a day among people living in developing countries.

Audrey Eyton's diet showed us that by boosting our fibre intake (by eating more wholemeal pasta and bread and whole-grain rice, potatoes with their skins on, pulses and beans) we could lose weight without feeling hungry.

As well as helping you to slim, fibre in your diet takes good care of your digestive system and keeps your bowels healthy. Most importantly for PMS sufferers, it keeps your blood sugar level stable, your moods on an even keel and your cravings in check.

Fibre reduces your cravings for sweet and fatty foods because it slows down and evens out both the rate at which sugar is released into your blood and the rate at which it is cleared away. The amount of sugar circulating in the blood is controlled by insulin, a hormone secreted by the pancreas, and the amount of fibre in your diet is thought to have an effect on the amount of insulin you produce. After eating apples, apple purée or apple juice, for example, your blood sugar level will rise. The fibre in the purée and in the solid apple will help the blood sugar level to return to normal, whereas, after drinking just the apple juice, which contains no fibre, your blood sugar level will drop below normal.

We should aim to eat 18 grams (about $\frac{3}{4}$ oz) of dietary fibre each day. The following table shows how much fibre different foods provide.

Where to get your fibre

	Percentage of fibre	Grams per portion		Percentage of fibre	Grams per portion
Breakfast cereals					
All Bran	26.7	11.3	Leeks	3.1	3.5
Bran Flakes	11.8	5.0	Avocados	2.0	2.8
Sultana Bran	10.6	4.5	Mushrooms	2.5	2.8
Muesli	7.4	4.2	Tomatoes	1.5	1.7
Weetabix	12.7	3.6			
Sugarpuffs	6.1	1.7	*Fruit*		
Special K	5.5	1.6	Dried figs	18.5	10.5
Cornflakes	3.0	0.8	Apricots		
			dried	24.0	6.8
Vegetables and pulses			stewed	8.9	10.0
Peas			Raspberries	7.4	8.4
fresh or frozen	8.0	9.1	Blackberries	7.3	8.3
dried split	11.9	6.7	Dried dates	8.7	4.9
tinned	7.9	11.2	Cherries	1.5	3.4
Haricot beans	25.4	7.2	Bananas	2.0	3.4
French beans	3.2	3.6	Oranges	1.5	2.5
Runner beans	3.4	3.9	Prunes	13.4	1.9
Kidney beans			*Bread*		
dried	25.0	7.1	Granary	6.8	4.8
canned	8.0	6.8	High bran	11.1	7.9
Baked beans	7.3	16.5	Wholemeal	8.5	6.0
Sweetcorn	5.7	5.7			
Baked potatoes	2.5	5.0	*Pasta and rice*		
Carrots	3.0	3.4	Wholewheat pasta	10.0	5.7
Parsnips	2.5	2.8			
Lentils	11.7	5.0	Brown rice	4.3	2.5
Spinach	6.3	7.1	White rice	2.4	1.4
Broccoli	4.1	4.6			
Spring greens	3.8	4.3			
Brussels sprouts	2.9	3.3			

Fats

We need a small amount of fat in our diet to provide us with certain vitamins and essential fatty acids, and also to make our food more tasty. But there are healthy and harmful fats, and it's the latter we should avoid.

Saturated fats are bad for us because high levels of them in the blood blocks and damages the arteries and impedes blood circulation, increasing the risk of cardio-vascular disease. There is also a lot of evidence that reducing fat in the diet lowers the symptoms of PMS.

Most of us are now aware of the risks of a very high-fat diet and the last 15 years have seen a dramatic change in the way many of us eat. Gone from most breakfast tables is the traditional egg and bacon fry-up, but most people are still eating too many processed foods, which can contain a lot of fat.

There is also a lot of confusion about why polyunsaturated fats are good for us. It is because they make the blood less 'sticky', which prevents it from attaching itself to the arterial walls and causing blockages. Hence their beneficial effect on your health – unless you eat so much of them that your weight becomes a health problem!

- *Saturated fat* is found mainly in animal products such as red meat and dairy products. This type of fat can raise blood cholesterol.
- *Monounsaturated fat* is found in olive oil. This has no effect on blood cholesterol and can be used in moderation.
- *Polyunsaturated fat* is found mainly in vegetable oils such as corn oil and sunflower oil, in polyunsaturated margarines and in oily fish. It can lower blood cholesterol when taken as part of a low-fat diet, but remember, polyunsaturated fats contain the same high number of calories as other fats, so it's wise to go easy on them.

Vitamins and minerals

We all need minerals and vitamins, but the general recommendation is that, with a few exceptions (old people living alone who don't eat properly; dieters eating well below their nutritional requirements; and pregnant women), we should obtain all our nutrients from the food we eat, and not from dietary supplements.

One reason for this is that supplements can upset the body's natural balance if you are getting your nutrients from different sources. Many vitamins and minerals, such as iron and zinc, compete with each other for absorption. Flooding the system with one will cause a deficiency of another and may upset some body processes, or create additional requirements. This could be as harmful as not eating enough vitamin-rich foods.

It is often impossible to tell whether you are getting enough vitamins and minerals because signs of deficiency take a long time to manifest themselves. They also tend to be very vague. Lethargy and depression, for example, could be symptomatic of a shortage of any number of vitamins. Furthermore, our individual requirements and our ability to absorb and utilize nutrients change all the time.

Try a change of diet before pumping yourself with supplements. It could be that all your nutritional requirements are met by eating properly. Only if your symptoms persist should you consider supplements, and only after discussing them with your GP first.

The best way to maximize your vitamin and mineral intake is to buy fresh foods and cook them properly. Stir-frying, steaming and microwaving are all excellent cooking methods which retain the nutrients in the food.

The main supplements used to treat PMS are vitamin B_6, calcium and magnesium and evening primrose oil.

Vitamin B_6

Vitamin B_6, 'the anti-PMS vitamin', is particularly useful for the relief of mood changes, breast discomfort and headaches. Good sources of vitamin B_6 include whole grains, meat, fish, avocados, bananas and nuts. It must be taken with vitamin B_2 (riboflavin) and magnesium (found in whole grains, green vegetables and nuts) in order to work properly. A standard vitamin B complex tablet may provide all you need to balance the B_6.

An increase in headaches, nausea and restless sleep can indicate that your dose of vitamin B_6 is too high and should be reduced. Although vitamin B_6 has brought relief to thousands of PMS sufferers, some experts are still sceptical about its use. A group of doctors in the *New England Journal of Medicine* warned that taking vitamin B_6 in excessive doses can cause nerve damage.

One theory about why vitamin B_6 deficiency is so common among women with PMS is that high levels of oestrogen deplete the vitamin. High levels of vitamin B_6 are also vital for the healthy functioning of the hypothalamus, the control centre of the menstrual cycle.

Dr Michael Brush recommends that vitamin B_6 treatment should be started three days before the onset of expected symptoms for maximum benefit.

Since women vary greatly in the amount of vitamin B_6 they need to obtain a good response to treatment, you should start with two 20 mg tablets with breakfast and two 20 mg tablets with your evening meal. If this dose does not appear to be having any effect, increase it to one 50 mg tablet twice daily. If it is still ineffectual, your doctor may suggest you increase it to 60 or 75 mg twice daily. But such an increase must be supervised by a doctor, and each dose level should be tried for one or two menstrual cycles before moving up to a larger dose.

Once you have established the correct dose of B_6 for you, continue with it for six to eight months before attempting to reduce the dose. After that, if there are no problems, gradually reduce the dose, by 25 to 50 mg, every four weeks. If your symptoms return, go back to the original effective dose.

Calcium and magnesium

A dose of these minerals in the ratio of two parts calcium to one part magnesium (usually 500 mg to 250 mg) has traditionally been recommended to treat premenstrual and menstrual cramps. However, Dr Michelle Harrison, a leading authority on PMS, recommends that doses should be varied according to the symptoms. For example:

- If you have premenstrual and menstrual cramps, but no other

symptoms, take two parts calcium to one part magnesium.
- For PMS without cramps, take one part calcium to two parts magnesium.
- For PMS cramps with other symptoms, take equal amounts of calcium and magnesium.

Evening primrose oil

Several studies have shown evening primrose oil to be effective for symptoms such as breast tenderness and swelling as well as emotional symptoms. It is one of the richest sources of the EFA gamma-linolenic acid (GLA), and corrects underlying essential fatty acid deficiency at source by supplying what the body needs, thereby reaching the root of the problem.

Evening primrose oil is usually prepared in capsules of 500 mg, to be taken twice daily throughout the month. If the first month's treatment is not successful, increase the dosage to six capsules a day during the second month, and maybe eight capsules a day during the third month if six do not appear to be enough.

Though allergic reactions to evening primrose oil are rare, they do occur occasionally. Also, if you have any form of epilepsy, *do not* take evening primrose oil without consulting your doctor as there is some evidence that it can make the condition worse.

Other helpful vitamins and minerals

- *Vitamin C* is particularly concerned with the growth and repair of the body cells and tissues. It also contributes to hormone production, helps us to fight stress and protects us from infection. It is widely available in fruit and vegetables.

- *Vitamin E* – the 'anti-ageing vitamin' – supplies oxygen to the muscles and helps in the regeneration of new skin. Supplements of vitamin E have been used to treat PMS in some women, especially those suffering from breast tenderness, as it is thought to help balance the body's metabolism. Vitamin E can be found in nuts, rice, avocados and oily fish.

- *Vitamin A* and *beta carotene*, which is turned into vitamin A in the body and may protect against cancer, are found in carrots, spinach, greens and liver. Taken with zinc, vitamin A is particularly recommended for PMS acne.

- *The B vitamins* include vitamin B_1 (thiamin), vitamin B_2 (riboflavin), vitamin B_3 (niacin), vitamin B_6, vitamin B_{12} and folic acid. They are vital for the nervous system and also help to keep your skin, hair, eyes, mouth and liver in good health. Good sources of B vitamins are oily fish, wholemeal pasta and brown rice.

- *Calcium* is essential for strong bones and is also known to help premenstrual and menstrual cramps. It is found in milk, cheese, spinach and fish with bones, such as whitebait and sprats.

- *Iron* – essential for growth, resistance to infection, and hormone production – is found in offal, shellfish, oily fish and many types of bread. Adequate supplies of vitamin C are needed to help with the absorption of iron.

- *Zinc* helps to build cells and keeps hormone production healthy. The best sources are meat and shellfish, although zinc is also included in some breakfast cereals.

- *Potassium* helps balance sodium in the body and enables the nerves and muscles to function. Good sources of potassium include baked potatoes, stewed rhubarb and oily fish.

5

Healthy eating plans

The NAPS PMS Eating Plan

Because we are all different, with our own individual needs, it is impossible to formulate an eating plan that will suit everyone's requirements, but the PMS Eating Plan of the National Association for Premenstrual Syndrome (NAPS) can be used as a guide. This diet aims to produce a sustained rise in blood glucose levels throughout the whole month. It will relieve many of the more severe symptoms of PMS and may be all the treatment that is required.

Breakfast (within half an hour of rising)
pure fruit juice or half a grapefruit
5 tablespoons high-fibre breakfast cereal
2 medium slices wholemeal bread spread with
polyunsaturated or low-fat spread and low- or reduced-sugar
marmalade
tea or coffee with low-fat milk

Mid-morning
1 digestive biscuit
tea or coffee with low-fat milk

Midday or evening meal
lean meat or fish
medium jacket potato
large helping of vegetables or salad
fresh fruit or tinned fruit in natural juice

Mid-afternoon
1 digestive biscuit

tea or coffee with low-fat milk

Evening or midday meal
vegetable soup
2 slices wholemeal bread as a sandwich with meat or fish and
salad
fresh fruit

Bedtime or late evening
4 high-fibre crackers spread with polyunsaturated margarine
small helping of cheese or lean meat
milky drink

This basic plan gives about 1400 calories, derived from high-fibre
sources. A daily allowance of 600 ml (1 pint) of skimmed or semi-
skimmed milk must be drunk daily to ensure an adequate calcium
intake.

Varying your diet
It is important to add variety to your diet. NAPS suggest the
following alternatives for cereals and fruit, for example:

Cereals
5 tablespoons All Bran
5 tablespoons Bran Flakes
4 tablespoons unsweetened muesli
1 Shredded Wheat
1 Weetabix
6 tablespoons porridge
1 medium slice wholemeal bread
75 g (3 oz) cooked brown rice
4 low-calorie high-fibre crispbreads
75 g (3 oz) cooked wholemeal pasta
1 digestive biscuit
3 Ryvita

Fruit
1 medium apple
1 medium eating or cooking apple
1 large peach
1 medium banana
1 medium pear
1 medium orange
1 thick slice fresh pineapple
2 large tangerines
10 large grapes
2 large dessert plums
2 large stewed prunes
175 g (6 oz) strawberries
175 g (6 oz) raspberries

Note
If you are going to be more energetic than usual, playing sports, gardening or spring cleaning, for example, you should make sure you increase your intake of carbohydrates.

Weight-watchers and the PMS diet

At first glance you may think the PMS diet will cause you to put on weight as its carbohydrate content is being stressed. This is not the case. Although you are being asked to increase the amount of unrefined carbohydrates you eat, you are also being advised to cut down or cut out sugars and sugary foods, and to reduce your intake of fats. This combination will help you to lose weight slowly.

- Keep a careful watch on your weight: by changing your eating habits, you may reduce your calorie intake to below what you need, thereby causing an unnecessary weight loss.
- Weigh yourself once a week, at the same time of day each time.
- If you need to lose weight, decrease the quantity of carbohydrates in your diet – eat smaller portions of pasta, rice and baked potatoes – but do not compensate by eating more fatty foods.
- If you do not need to lose weight, but discover that you are

losing it anyway, increase the amount of carbohydrate in your meals.

The 1000 calories a day slimmers' eating plan

Breakfast
pure fruit juice or half a grapefruit
5 tablespoons high-fibre breakfast cereal
1 medium slice wholemeal bread with a scraping of low-fat
spread and low- or reduced-sugar marmalade
tea or coffee with low-fat milk

Mid-morning
1 serving fresh fruit
tea or coffee with low-fat milk

Midday or evening meal
lean meat or fish
medium jacket potato
large helping vegetables or salad
1 serving fresh fruit or tinned fruit in natural juice

Mid-afternoon
1 serving fresh fruit

Evening or midday meal
Vegetable soup
1 slice wholemeal bread or 3 Ryvita with meat or fish and
salad
1 serving fresh fruit

Bedtime or late evening snack
2 high-fibre crackers with small helping of cheese or lean
meat
milky drink

Daily allowance: 600 ml (1 pint) skimmed milk and 25 g (1 oz) polyunsaturated margarine

Points to remember

- The symptoms of PMS get worse when you skip meals, so eat regularly – every three hours.
- If you are not used to a diet that is high in fibre, start gently when introducing it. If you don't, you'll suffer from bloating, flatulence, wind and possibly stomach cramps.
- When you change to this type of diet you need to increase your fluid intake. If you don't you are likely to become constipated. Drink six to eight glasses of water a day, and try substituting herb teas for tea and coffee.
- If you are on a medically prescribed diet for any reason, talk to your doctor and dietician to see if your present diet can be adapted to conform to the diet for PMS.
- If you are a diabetic you should already be on a high-fibre diet, but do not change the prescribed carbohydrate portions without seeing your dietician first.
- Some people think they are getting all the right nutrients because they are using supplements. It is very important to be aware of the fact that whole, fresh foods, fresh fruit and vegetable juices and unpolluted water provide the foundation for a well-rounded diet.
- A few women are allergic to wheat and other grain products and, as allergies can be aggravated premenstrually, these women may find that their PMS appears to get worse when they eat certain foods. PMS is also sometimes linked to gut dysbiosis (candida). If you suffer from tiredness, thrush, bloating and food intolerances, you should seek specific help from a dietician who will be able to advise you on a low yeast, low sugar diet. However, most women do not suffer from these problems and, as this is a separate issue from PMS, you should not be wary of following the guidelines in this book.
- Healthy snacks include low-fat digestive biscuits, bananas, sandwiches with salad or lean-meat fillings, rice cakes, toast,

teacakes and malt loaf with low-fat spread. Foods made with white flour, such as cakes and biscuits, sweets and chocolate are not recommended as part of your normal diet and should be kept for an occasional treat.

- In addition to avoiding processed foods, refined sugar and white-flour foods which are high in salt content, you should try to keep alcohol, caffeine, chocolate, nicotine and dairy products to a minimum, especially when you are experiencing PMS symptoms.

Shopping and eating out

Shopping for healthy food needn't be expensive. And there's no need to make a special trip to a health-food store. Wholemeal bread, wholewheat pasta and brown rice are as easy to buy from your local supermarket as the refined, 'white' varieties.

- Make the most of seasonal vegetables, for value-for-money shopping.
- Buy more tinned oily fish and fewer processed meats and sausages.
- Yoghurt is cheaper than cream, and much healthier. The same goes for sunflower and olive oil spreads, as alternatives to butter.

Eating out on the PMS diet shouldn't be a problem once you understand the rules. For example, choose:

salad instead of a rich and creamy starter
grilled meat or fish rather than fried
baked potatoes or rice instead of chips
pasta instead of pizza
tomato sauces based on olive oil rather than cream
fruit desserts instead of ice cream or cheese.

Take-aways are still OK if you choose sensibly. For example, you could pick an Indian Tandoori or chicken tikka (without the creamy sauce), with salad and wholemeal bread instead of a rich ghee-based curry, or a baked potato instead of fish and chips.

You can widen the variety in your diet while still eating healthily. The recipes included in Part 2 are intended to whet your appetite and show you that fresh fruit and vegetables, salads and high-fibre foods can be exciting and enjoyable. I have tried to choose dishes which you could serve to family and friends. Your PMS diet should not isolate you, but improve the health of the whole family.

PART 2

Recipes

Note: measures are given in both metric and imperial (the conversions are *approximate*, having been rounded up or down). Use either system – not a mixture of the two – in any recipe. All spoon measures are level unless stated otherwise.

SALADS

Carrot, orange and tomato salad

Serves 4

This colourful salad is rich in vitamin C and beta carotene, which is
made into vitamin A by the body.

> *2 large slicing tomatoes*
> *2 large oranges*
> *2 large carrots, peeled*
> *lettuce leaves*

DRESSING
150 ml/ ¼ pint olive oil
5 tablespoons sunflower oil
juice and grated rind of 1
   orange

1 tablespoon wine vinegar
1 teaspoon mild mustard
1 teaspoon caster sugar
salt and milled pepper

Skin and seed the tomatoes and cut them into petals. Peel the
oranges with a knife and cut into segments. Coarsely grate the
carrots.

Make up the dressing by combining all the ingredients.

Arrange the fruit and vegetables on lettuce leaves in individual
bowls. Dress before serving or pass the dressing separately.

Winter salad with cheese

Serves 6

The peppers in this salad are rich in vitamin C and beta carotene.
Cheese, although an animal fat, can still be enjoyed in moderation
and is a good source of calcium.

> *2 green peppers*
> *2 red peppers*
> *250 g/8 oz low-fat Cheddar cheese*

DRESSING

> *150 ml/¼ pint olive oil*
> *2 tablespoons wine vinegar*
> *1 clove garlic, crushed*
> *1 teaspoon mild mustard*
> *salt and freshly milled pepper*

Cut the peppers and the cheese into fine strips. Chill in separate
containers and mix together just before serving. Toss in the dressing
just before your guests sit down.

Cheese, cucumber, tomato and orange salad

Serves 6

225 g/8 oz mature low-fat cheese, cut into cubes
2 large slicing tomatoes, skinned, seeded and cut into chunks
1 small cucumber, seeded and cut into chunks
1 dozen anchovies, rolled, to garnish

DRESSING
150 ml/¼ pint olive oil
juice and finely grated rind of
   1 orange
1 teaspoon mild mustard

salt and milled pepper
1 clove garlic, crushed
   (optional)
1 teaspoon caster sugar

Put the dressing ingredients in a screw-topped jar and shake well.
   Mix the salad ingredients in a large bowl and chill.
   Dress the salad just before serving. Garnish with the anchovies.

Spinach, bacon and avocado salad

Serves 4

Avocados are a rich source of vitamin B_6, vitamin C, vitamin E, iron and zinc. The spinach also contains vitamins and calcium and adds fibre to this tasty salad.

75 g/3 oz ready-prepared
*   baby spinach leaves*
6 rashers rindless bacon
1 avocado pear
juice of half a lemon

2 tablespoons olive or walnut
*   oil*
1/2 teaspoon Dijon mustard
freshly ground black pepper

Arrange the spinach in a salad bowl.

Grill the bacon until crisp. Cool and chop into small pieces. Add to the spinach leaves.

Peel and remove the stone from the avocado. Dice the flesh and dip into the lemon juice to prevent discoloration. Drain and add to the salad.

Whisk together 2 teaspoons lemon juice, the oil, mustard and black pepper. Pour this dressing over the salad, toss lightly and serve.

Cashew nut and orange salad

A special occasion salad! Nuts contain vitamin E and fibre, and the orange beta carotene and vitamin C. Watercress is also a good source of vitamin C and calcium.

> *100 g/4 oz unsalted cashew nuts*
> *4 large tomatoes, peeled and sliced*
> *1 small head fennel, sliced finely*
> *1 lettuce heart, chopped*
> *1 small bunch watercress, trimmed and washed*

DRESSING

> *1 teaspoon mild mustard*
> *2 tablespoons orange juice*
> *grated rind of 1 orange*
> *110 ml/4 fl oz olive oil*
> *sea salt*

Mix all the salad ingredients together.

Combine the mustard, orange juice and orange rind and slowly stir in the olive oil so that the sauce is well blended. Season to taste with sea salt.

Toss the salad with the dressing just before serving.

Chicory, red pepper and orange salad

Serves 4

This recipe is high in vitamins A and C and garlic, which has antibacterial qualities (useful if you suffer from PMS as infections worsen the symptoms).

> *2 heads chicory*
> *1 red pepper*
> *4 large sticks celery*
> *1 large orange*

DRESSING

> *4 tablespoons olive or sunflower oil*
> *2 tablespoons wine vinegar*
> *1 teaspoon mild mustard*
> *1 clove garlic, crushed*
> *freshly ground black pepper*

Cut each chicory head in half lengthways and then thinly slice it.

Cut the pepper into strips.

Chop the celery.

Remove the rind and pith from the orange, then cut the flesh into quarters lengthways and thinly slice it.

In a salad bowl mix together the chicory, pepper, celery and orange.

Beat the remaining ingredients together to make the dressing and fold them into the salad.

Greek salad

Serves 4

This salad is rich in vitamins A and C and calcium.

2 large slicing tomatoes, cut
  into segments
half an onion, sliced finely
half a green pepper, sliced
  thinly
10 cm/4 inch piece of
  cucumber, peeled and
  sliced

6–8 black or green olives
125 g/4 oz feta cheese (rinsed
  briefly if too salty)
pinch of dried oregano
5 tablespoons good quality
  olive oil
salt

Mix all the ingredients in a bowl and serve.

Green salad

Serves 4

1 small lettuce heart
1 small crisp lettuce
a quarter of a cucumber,
  sliced

4 spring onions
1 small bunch watercress
1 tablespoon olive oil

DRESSING

1–2 tablespoons lemon juice
large pinch mustard powder
1 teaspoon clear honey
1 clove garlic, crushed
black pepper

Prepare the salad ingredients and refrigerate. Then, just before serving, toss in the olive oil.

For the dressing, mix the remaining ingredients together and toss into the salad.

Serve immediately.

Guacamole

Serves 4

A very good anti-PMS dish – avocados are rich in iron and vitamin B_6, vitamin E, vitamin C and zinc.

2 large ripe avocados	*1 small bunch fresh coriander*
2 medium tomatoes	*leaves*
juice of half a lemon	*splash of Tabasco sauce*
1 clove garlic, crushed	*salt and pepper*

Combine all the ingredients in a food processor until smooth and creamy. Turn into a serving dish and place the avocado stone in the centre to prevent the mixture from turning brown.

Serve immediately as a pre-dinner snack with fresh, raw vegetables, such as carrot sticks, strips of red and green pepper and lengths of celery.

Tomato, mozzarella, avocado and rocket salad

Allow a tomato, half an avocado, a small piece of mozzarella cheese and a small bunch of rocket leaves per person. Slice the avocados, tomatoes and cheese and mix with the peppery rocket leaves. Dress the salad with olive oil, balsamic vinegar and salt if required and serve immediately.

FRUIT

Exotic fruit salad

Serves 12

1 pineapple
1 mango
2 nectarines
2 melons
3 kiwi fruit
2 peaches

6 apricots
6 lychees
3 passion fruit
rind of 1 orange, sliced, to
    garnish

Cut the pineapple in half. Using a sharp knife, peel and core it. Cut into slices, then into even-sized fan-shaped pieces.

Peel the mango with a potato-peeler. Carve the flesh away from the stone as neatly as possible, then cut into tidy pieces.

Cut the nectarines in half and pit but do not skin them. Cut into crescents.

Halve and seed the melons and scoop out the flesh with a melon-baller.

Peel the kiwi fruit and cut into thinnish discs about 2.5 mm ($\frac{1}{8}$ inch) thick.

Skin the peaches, having first dipped them quickly into a pan of boiling water, then cut them in half and take out the stones. Cut into crescents, then in half again.

Halve and pit the apricots and skin and halve the lychees.

Chill all these ingredients well for 2–4 hours.

Just before serving, cut the passion fruit in half, scoop out the pulp and mix with the other fruit. Decorate with strips of orange rind.

Melon with mango and kiwi fruit

Serves 2

Mangoes are rich in vitamins A and C, and kiwi fruit in vitamin C.

> *1 melon*
> *2 tablespoons lemon juice*
> *1 small mango*
> *1 kiwi fruit*

Cut the melon in half and scoop out the seeds. Pour a little lemon juice into each half.

Peel the mango and cut out wedges of the flesh. Cut each wedge into smaller segments.

Peel the kiwi fruit. Cut into discs, then into smaller pieces.

Toss the two kiwi fruit and mango together in a basin with the remaining lemon juice. Pile into the melon halves. Cover with plastic film and chill for 4 hours.

Citrus fruit salad

Serves 4

2 pink grapefruit
4 medium oranges
2 tablespoons clear honey
2 bananas

Peel the grapefruit and oranges and remove the pith. Divide the fruit into segments. If the grapefruit segments are large, cut them in half.

Put the fruit in a bowl. Fold in the honey and chill for 15 minutes.

Peel and slice the bananas and fold them into the rest of the fruit. Serve immediately.

Pineapple and dried fruit salad

Serves 4

This a tasty high-fibre dessert. Note that the dried fruit needs to be soaked in advance.

125 g/4¹/₂ oz dried whole apricots
8 prunes
25 g/1 oz dried apple rings

300 ml/¹/₂ pint orange or pineapple juice
1 small pineapple
2 tablespoons chopped toasted hazelnuts to garnish

Soak the apricots, prunes and apple rings in the orange or pineapple juice for 8 hours.

Peel and slice the pineapple and chop up the slices, removing the cores. Mix the pineapple with the dried fruit and juice and chill for a further hour.

Put the fruit salad in serving bowls, scatter the toasted hazelnuts on top and serve at once.

Rice ring with peaches

Serves 4

The rice in this dish is an excellent form of fibre.

175 g/6 oz long-grain brown rice
600 ml/1 pint apple juice
1/4 teaspoon ground nutmeg
11 g/1/2 oz sachet agar (the vegetarian alternative to gelatine)

4 tablespoons warm water
450 g/1 lb carton natural yoghurt
4 peaches

Put the rice in a saucepan with the apple juice and nutmeg. Bring to the boil. Cover the pan and simmer for 30–40 minutes or until the rice is soft. Drain off excess juice if necessary.

In a small pan, soak the agar in the warm water and then melt it on a low heat and stir it into the rice. Leave the mixture to cool. Mix in the yoghurt.

Put one peach in a bowl and pour boiling water over it. Leave for 2 minutes, then drain it and peel off the skin. Stone and slice the peach.

Lay the peach slices in the bottom of an oiled 900 ml/1 1/2 pint ring mould in a cool place for 2 hours to set.

Just before serving, scald, skin and slice the remaining peaches. Turn out the rice mould and fill the centre with the sliced peaches.

Fruit and nut salad

Serves 4

1 peach, stoned and sliced
2 oranges, peeled and
  segmented
225 g/8 oz fresh pineapple,
  peeled and chopped

175 g/6 oz seedless green
  grapes
25 g/1 oz Brazil nuts,
  chopped
juice of 1 orange

Wash and prepare all the fruit. Arrange a circle of the peach and orange slices on 4 plates.

Mix together the pineapple, grapes and nuts and pile up in the middle of the peach and orange circles.

Spoon over the orange juice.

Cottage cheese and fruit platter

Serves 4

You can vary the fruit according to season with this versatile dish.

100 g/4 oz seedless green
  grapes
2 passion fruit or 2 fresh figs,
  halved
100 g/4 oz raspberries

100 g/4 oz black cherries
1 orange
1 star fruit
225 g/8 oz cottage cheese

Wash all the fruit. Peel and slice the orange and slice the star fruit, but leave the raspberries whole and the cherries on their stems.

Divide the cottage cheese into 4 and pile up in the centre of 4 individual plates. Arrange the fruit in attractive clusters around the cheese.

PULSES

Hummus

Serves 4–6

Hummus is a classic Greek dip which is full of goodness. It is made from chick peas, which actually rival lean meat as a source of protein. They also contain more calcium than any other bean, several minerals and some vitamin C. Remember to soak them in advance. Tahini is a paste made from sesame seeds, which are rich in calcium and vitamin E.

175 g/6 oz chick peas, picked clean and soaked overnight
2 cloves garlic
2 tablespoons tahini (sesame paste)
juice of 1½ lemons
1½ teaspoons ground cumin

4 tablespoons vegetable oil – choose one that is high in polyunsaturates or monosaturates
salt and black pepper
1–2 tablespoons olive oil and a little cayenne pepper or paprika to garnish

Rinse the chick peas. Cover with plenty of water in a large pan, bring to the boil and skim until clear. Cover and cook until soft. (In a pressure cooker they will take 15–20 minutes, otherwise a little over 1 hour, according to their age.)

Strain the chick peas, reserving the cooking liquid.

Place the remaining ingredients and 300 ml/½ pint of the cooking liquid in a food processor or liquidizer and blend until grainy and of a runny consistency. (You will probably have to divide up the ingredients and process them in two batches.) If too dry, add more liquid and then adjust the seasoning and blend it in briefly.

Pour the hummus into a shallow bowl and sprinkle the oil and the cayenne pepper or paprika decoratively on top before serving.

Chick pea casserole

Serves 4

225 g/8 oz chick peas, picked
   clean and soaked overnight
150 ml/¼ pint olive oil
1 large onion, sliced thinly

2 cloves garlic, chopped
2 carrots, scraped and sliced
3 tablespoons tomato purée
salt and black pepper

Wash and strain the chick peas. Cover with plenty of water in a pan, bring to the boil and skim until clear. Cover and cook until almost soft, about an hour (15–20 minutes if using a pressure cooker).

Drain the chick peas, reserving 450 ml/³⁄₄ pint of their cooking liquid. Use this to dilute the tomato purée.

Heat the olive oil and fry the onion and garlic until a light golden-brown. Add the chick peas, diluted tomato purée and the rest of the ingredients. Mix well, cover and cook for 40 minutes or until the sauce thickens and the chick peas are very soft.

This casserole can be served at room temperature, like all olive oil-based dishes.

Cannellini bean soup

Serves 6

225 g/8 oz cannellini or
    haricot beans, picked clean
    and soaked overnight
1 medium onion, sliced finely
2 carrots, sliced thinly
2 small sticks celery, sliced
    thinly
400 g/14 oz can chopped
    tomatoes

1 teaspoon tomato purée
1 tablespoon each dried
    oregano and thyme
150 ml/¼ pint olive oil
2 tablespoons chopped fresh
    parsley
salt and black pepper

Wash and drain the beans. Cover with water in a large pan, boil for 3 minutes and drain again, discarding the water. (This step makes the beans digestible.)

Return the beans to the pan with 900 ml/1½ pints water and the rest of the ingredients, apart from the salt and chopped parsley. Cover and cook for about 1 hour, or until the beans are soft but not disintegrating. (If using a pressure cooker, which is ideal for this dish, cook for 6–7 minutes under full pressure.)

Add the salt and parsley and simmer for 5 more minutes before serving.

Tuna and haricot bean salad

Serves 4

Haricot beans contain iron, magnesium and zinc. Tuna is excellent for combating PMS because it is an oily fish containing zinc, vitamin E and calcium.

1 400 g/14 oz can haricot
  beans
200 g/7 oz can tuna fish,
  drained and flaked
5 medium tomatoes
4 tablespoons chopped fresh
  parsley

4 tablespoons reduced-fat
  mayonnaise
2 tablespoons natural yoghurt
juice of 1 lemon
1 clove garlic, crushed
freshly ground black pepper

Mix the tuna with the haricot beans.

Chop 3 of the tomatoes and mix these and half the parsley into the tuna and beans.

Mix together the mayonnaise, yoghurt, lemon juice, garlic and pepper. Fold this dressing into the salad.

Arrange the salad on a serving plate. Garnish it with the remaining tomatoes, cut into wedges or slices, and scatter the remaining parsley over the top.

Lamb in the pot with beans

Serves 4

225 g/8 oz cannellini beans
450 g/1 lb lean boneless lamb
4 large sticks celery, chopped
1 large onion, sliced thinly
1 tablespoon chopped fresh
  thyme or 1 teaspoon dried
  thyme
2 teaspoons chopped fresh
  rosemary or 1 teaspoon
  dried rosemary

600 ml/1 pint chicken stock
300 ml/½ pint tomato juice
dash of Tabasco sauce
2 teaspoons paprika
1 clove garlic, crushed

Put the beans in a saucepan. Cover with water, bring to the boil and simmer, covered, for 10 minutes. Remove from heat and leave to soak for 2 hours. Drain.

Preheat the oven to Gas Mark 4/180 °C/350 °F.

Cut the lamb into 2 cm/1 inch dice.

Layer the beans, lamb, celery, onion and herbs in a deep casserole.

Mix the rest of the ingredients together and pour them over the lamb and beans.

Cover the casserole and cook in the oven for 2 hours, or until the beans and lamb are really tender.

Tomato and lentil soup

Serves 4

Lentils are rich in vitamin B_6, iron, phosphorus and zinc. There are four main varieties: red split lentils, green lentils, brown lentils and 'blue' lentils.

700 g/1½ lb ripe tomatoes
3 tablespoons sunflower oil
1 large onion, chopped finely
1 clove garlic, chopped finely
100 g/4 oz split red lentils
2 tablespoons chopped fresh parsley
1 tablespoon chopped fresh thyme or 1 teaspoon dried thyme

1 tablespoon chopped fresh marjoram or 1 teaspoon dried marjoram
600 ml/1 pint vegetable stock
a pinch of sea salt
freshly ground black pepper

Scald, skin and chop the tomatoes.

Heat the oil in a saucepan on a low heat. Fry the onion and garlic until soft.

Add the tomatoes, lentils and herbs. Stir for 2 minutes or until the tomatoes are soft. Mash the mixture with a fork. Pour in the stock, bring to the boil and season. Cover the pan and simmer for 45 minutes.

Baguette filled with cannellini beans and sardines

Serves 4

Sardines are rich in calcium and fish oil.

1 wholemeal French stick
3 tablespoons sunflower oil
1 large onion, sliced thinly
1 teaspoon paprika
¼ teaspoon chilli powder
400 g/14 oz cannellini
   beans, drained

2 120 g/4½ oz cans sardines in
   brine, drained
juice of 1 lemon
4 tablespoons chopped fresh
   parsley

Cut the French stick into 4 equal pieces. Slit them down the side and remove most of the crumb, leaving just the shells.

Preheat the oven to Gas Mark 6/200 °C/400 °F.

Heat the oil in a saucepan on a low heat. Stir in the onion, paprika and chilli powder and cook gently until the onion is soft.

Mix in the beans, sardines, lemon juice and parsley.

Fill the bread cases with the beans and sardines. Wrap individually in foil and place on a baking sheet. Bake in the oven for 20 minutes.

VEGETABLES

Carrot and courgette stew

Serves 4

225 g/½ lb carrots, sliced
  5 mm/¼ inch thick
450 g/1 lb small courgettes,
  sliced 5 mm/¼ inch thick
100 g/4 oz butter

4 tomatoes, peeled and
  chopped
salt, pepper and sugar
extra knob of butter
parsley, chopped

Blanch the carrots in boiling salted water for 3 minutes. Add the courgettes and boil for a further 3–5 minutes, until the vegetables are half-cooked. Drain well.

Melt the butter in large heavy frying-pan. Add the carrots and courgettes. Cook gently, stirring often, for 10 minutes.

Add the tomatoes and reduce to a thick buttery sauce.

Season with salt, pepper and sugar to taste. Stir in the extra knob of butter, sprinkle with parsley and serve.

Curried carrots

Serves 4

700 g/1½ lb carrots, sliced
  diagonally
1 small onion, chopped
1 clove garlic, chopped
50 g/2 oz butter
2 rounded tablespoons flour
1 tablespoon curry powder
1 eating apple, cored and
  diced

225 g/8 oz low-fat fromage
  frais
either 75 g/3 oz raisins and
50 g/2 oz blanched split
almonds, or 3 hard-boiled
eggs, quartered
salt and pepper

Cook the carrots in 25 mm/1 inch of boiling, salted water. Drain, reserving the cooking liquor.

Stew the onion and garlic in butter until soft. Stir in flour and curry powder. Moisten with the carrot liquor.

Add the apple and fromage frais. Simmer for about 15 minutes.

Stir in the carrots and reheat, adding the raisins and almonds or the eggs.

Serve in a ring of buttered boiled rice.

Ratatouille

Serves 4

1 tablespoon olive oil
1 onion, chopped
2 cloves garlic, crushed
1 medium aubergine, diced
4 courgettes, sliced
2 red peppers, deseeded and
  diced

400 g/14 oz can tomatoes
1 bay-leaf
sprig of fresh thyme
50–75 g/2–3 oz pine kernels or
  sunflower seeds
salt and pepper

Heat the oil in a pan and gently fry the onion for a few minutes.

Add the garlic, aubergine, courgettes and peppers. Cook for 10 minutes, stirring occasionally.

Add the tomatoes and herbs and cook gently for 40 minutes, until the vegetables are fairly soft.

Stir in the pine kernels or sunflower seeds, season well and serve immediately.

Stuffed aubergines

Serves 4

The apricots in this stuffing provide fibre, vitamin B$_6$, magnesium and some calcium and iron.

2 small aubergines	*$^1/_2$ teaspoon ground coriander*
225 g/8 oz red split lentils	*75 g/3 oz dried apricots,*
2 teaspoons olive oil	*chopped*
1 small onion, finely chopped	*2 tablespoons apple juice*
$^1/_2$ teaspoon ground cumin	*1 tablespoon soy sauce*

Halve the aubergines and scoop out the flesh. Retain the shells.

Cover the lentils with water. Bring to the boil, cover and simmer for 15–20 minutes. Drain, and reserve any excess liquid.

Heat the oil over a moderate heat and gently cook the onion, cumin and coriander for 5 minutes. Stir in the aubergine flesh and drained lentils and cook for 5–8 minutes. Add the apricots, apple juice, soy sauce and 3 tablespoons of stock or water. Cook for a further 5 minutes. Check the seasoning.

Fill the aubergine shells with the cooked mixture. Cover and bake in a preheated oven at Gas Mark 5/190 °C/375 °F for 45 minutes.

Aubergine and mushroom rice

Serves 4

225 g/8 oz long-grain brown
    rice
2 teaspoons olive oil
1 large onion, chopped
1 large clove garlic, crushed
1 large aubergine, diced
100 g/4 oz mushrooms,
    quartered

2 teaspoons chopped fresh
    marjoram
2 teaspoons chopped fresh
    thyme
1 teaspoon paprika
25 g/1 oz wholemeal flour
300 ml/½ pint skimmed milk
1 tablespoon soy sauce

Place the rice in a pan with 600 ml/1 pint boiling water. Bring to the boil, cover and simmer for 25 minutes. Drain the rice and transfer to a large casserole or ovenproof dish.

Heat the oil and gently fry the onion and garlic for 5 minutes. Add the aubergine and mushrooms and cook for a further 10 minutes.

Add the marjoram, thyme, paprika and flour and cook for 2–3 minutes. Stir in the milk and simmer for 5 minutes. Add the soy sauce and check the seasoning.

Spoon the aubergine mixture on top of the rice. Cover and bake in a preheated oven at Gas Mark 4/180 °C/350 °F for 30 minutes. Serve hot.

Tomatoes stuffed with goat's cheese, nuts and garlic

Serves 4

4 large tomatoes
50 g/2 oz chopped walnuts
25 g/1 oz wholemeal
  breadcrumbs
2 cloves garlic, crushed
50 g/2 oz goat's cheese

1 tablespoon chopped fresh
  herbs
1 free-range egg, beaten
sea salt and freshly ground
  black pepper

Trim the stem end of each tomato, then turn upside down and cut one third off the base of each one. (They will be cooked and served stem-side down, as this makes for a steadier base.)

Scoop out all the pulp, discarding the seeds where possible but reserving the flesh in a bowl. Place the tomato shells upside down to drain while the filling is prepared.

Put the walnuts, breadcrumbs and garlic in a bowl, then mash in the cheese. Add the herbs and blend in the egg. Season to taste with salt and pepper. Stir the chopped tomato pulp into the mixture and ensure that everything is well mixed.

Fill the tomato shells with the mixture and stand them in a shallow baking dish. Bake at Gas Mark 8/230 °C/450 °F for 5–8 minutes, so that the filling is cooked but the tomatoes have not had time to collapse or split. Serve at once.

Vegetable mixed grill

Serves 4

8 medium open-cap mushrooms
4 tomatoes
4 small courgettes
1 medium aubergine, weighing about 350 g/12 oz

MARINADE
110 ml/4 fl oz olive or
  sunflower oil
juice of 1 lemon
2 tablespoons tomato purée
2 teaspoons paprika

a pinch of chilli powder
2 tablespoons chopped fresh
  thyme or 2 teaspoons dried
  thyme

Trim the stalks of the mushrooms, leaving only about 5 mm/¼ inch.
Halve the tomatoes crossways.
Cut each courgette in half lengthways.
Cut the aubergine into 8 slices of equal thickness.
Mix together the ingredients for the marinade. Turn the mushrooms, courgettes and aubergines in the marinade and leave them for 30 minutes.
Just before cooking, brush some of the marinade over the tomatoes.
Heat the grill to high. Grill the courgettes for 2 minutes on each side, the aubergines for about 1½ minutes on each side, the mushrooms for 1½ minutes each side, and the tomatoes, cut-side up only, for 2 minutes.
Arrange the cooked vegetables attractively on a serving plate and serve.

MEAT

Fillet of beef salad

Serves 4

175 g/6 oz fillet steak
1 small cauliflower
175 g/6 oz broccoli
100 g/4 oz French beans, topped and tailed
225 g/8 oz cherry tomatoes

DRESSING
3 tablespoons olive oil
1 tablespoon wine vinegar
1 teaspoon Dijon mustard
1 teaspoon grated fresh
  horseradish

1 garlic clove, crushed
1 tablespoon fresh chopped
  chives

Trim the fillet steak. Grill it on a stove-top griddle (or fry it in a heavy pan at high heat) for 6 minutes. Leave to get completely cold.

Cut the cauliflower and broccoli into florets. Cook in boiling water for about 5 minutes, until they are half-tender. Refresh under running cold water and drain well.

Cook the beans for 2 minutes, refresh under running cold water and drain well.

Wash the tomatoes and remove any stalks.

Mix together the ingredients for the dressing – except the chives – very well. Use a tiny wire whisk if you have one.

Cut the steak into strips the size of your little finger. Mix them in a large bowl with the cauliflower, broccoli, tomatoes and beans.

Add the dressing and half the chives and stir gently.

Pile the salad into a serving dish and garnish with the remaining chives.

71

Lamb and peanut burgers

Serves 4

8 teaspoons peanut butter,
  chilled
450 g/1 lb minced lean lamb
1 medium onion, peeled and
  finely chopped
40 g/1½ oz finely chopped
  roasted peanuts
½ teaspoon dried mixed herbs

salt and freshly ground
  pepper
a little flour
oil for shallow frying
4 wholemeal hamburger rolls,
  toasted
2 tomatoes, sliced, and sprigs
  of parsley, to garnish

Form the peanut butter into 8 balls, put them on a plate and keep chilled.

Mix together the lamb, onion, peanuts, herbs and a little salt and pepper in a bowl. Divide into 4 equal portions and with floured hands shape each into a flat round burger.

Heat a little oil in a frying-pan and fry the burgers over moderate heat for 6–8 minutes on each side, or until cooked through.

Drain and serve in the toasted rolls, garnished with the peanut butter balls, tomato slices and parsley sprigs.

Chicken and mushroom hotpot

Serves 6

sunflower or olive oil for
    frying
50 g/2 oz diced bacon
a 1.5 kg/3 lb chicken, divided
    into 6 pieces
175 g/6 oz small onions,
    peeled
175 g/6 oz button mushrooms
1 clove garlic, crushed
2 tablespoons wholemeal flour

350 ml/12 fl oz strong chicken
    stock
1 can baked beans
1 bay-leaf
2 sprigs parsley
2 sprigs rosemary
salt and freshly ground black
    pepper

Heat the oil in a flameproof casserole or heavy pan and fry the bacon until pale golden. Remove with a slotted spoon.

Add the chicken pieces to the pan, brown quickly on all sides, then remove.

Fry the onions and mushrooms, stirring frequently, until the onions are golden.

Spoon off about half the fat, add the garlic and flour and stir over a low heat until the flour begins to brown. Then gradually add the stock and beans and bring to the boil, stirring constantly.

Return the chicken and bacon to the pan and add the bay-leaf, parsley and one sprig of rosemary. Season lightly with salt and pepper and bring back to boiling point. Stir, then reduce the heat and cover. Simmer for 45 minutes.

Remove the herbs, adjust the seasoning if necessary and serve garnished with the remaining sprig of rosemary.

Chicken breasts with red pepper sauce

Serves 4

4 chicken breasts, skinned
  and boned
3 tablespoons very finely
  shredded white of leek
2 tablespoons very finely
  shredded carrot

2 tablespoons chopped fresh
  mint
salt and freshly ground black
  pepper
1 bunch watercress to garnish

RED PEPPER SAUCE
1 red pepper
1 onion, chopped
1 tablespoon sunflower oil
2 tomatoes, peeled and
  deseeded

1 garlic clove
1 bouquet garni
salt and pepper

First make the sauce. Grill the pepper, skin side uppermost, until black all over. Skin it and cut the flesh into strips.

Cook the onion in the oil until it is just beginning to soften. Add the tomatoes, red pepper, garlic and bouquet garni. Stir in 6 tablespoons of water, bring the sauce to the boil and season with salt and pepper. Cover the pan, reduce the heat and cook the sauce for 20 minutes.

Remove the bouquet garni and liquidize the sauce until smooth. Then push it through a sieve into a clean container and chill.

Remove any fat from the chicken breasts.

Mix the leek, carrot and mint together and season them. Put this stuffing between the main part of the breasts and the loose fillet. Wrap each breast in a piece of cling film and poach the chicken breasts in simmering water for 15 minutes.

Remove the breasts from the pan, unwrap and leave to become completely cold.

Flood the base of 4 large plates with the red pepper sauce. Put a chicken breast on each plate and garnish with watercress leaves. Serve with brown rice, or potatoes in their skins.

Chicken, noodle and melon salad with peanut cream sauce

Serves 6–8

Fruit can be used in a main course like this one. The peanut dressing in this dish makes it a treat (for special occasions only, as salty peanuts eaten in quantity may cause premenstrual bloating if you are prone to it).

2 chickens
1 leek
1 carrot
1 onion
1 bouquet garni
half a lemon

300 g/12 oz noodles or
    vermicelli
salt
2 tablespoons groundnut oil
2 small melons
spring onions to garnish

PEANUT SAUCE
half a jar smooth peanut
    butter
a teacup of chicken stock
    reserved from cooking the
    chickens
2 tablespoons soy sauce
2 cloves garlic, crushed

2 2.5 cm/1 inch pieces ginger
    root, grated
1 tablespoon caster sugar
1 tablespoon lemon juice
2 dashes Tabasco sauce
300 ml/$\frac{1}{2}$ pint single cream

Wash the chickens under cold running water. Peel and roughly chop the leek, carrot and onion. Bring the vegetables, spices, lemon and herbs to the boil in a large pan with 1.2 litres/2 pints water. Reduce the heat and simmer for 15 minutes. Put in the chickens and simmer until the thighs are just tender (about 50 minutes to an hour).

Remove the chickens and cool. Strain the stock into a second pan, reserving 600 ml/1 pint. Boil the rest rapidly to reduce to about 300 ml (a teacupful). Cool and retain for the peanut sauce.

Before the chickens are completely cold, strip the meat from the carcasses and carve into slices.

Boil the noodles or vermicelli according to the instructions on the packet. Drain and turn into a bowl, stir in a couple of tablespoons of groundnut oil and leave to cool.

Peel the melons, seed them and cut into neat pieces.

Using a blender, or a food processor fitted with plastic blade, blend together all the dressing ingredients except the cream. Scrape the mixture out of the blender and stir in the cream to form a sauce.

To assemble the salad, arrange the cold noodles on a large platter and lay the chicken and melon on top. Dribble over a little of the sauce and serve the rest in a sauce-boat. Garnish with strips of spring onion if desired.

Stir-fried chicken with cashews

Serves 4

450 g/1 lb boneless, skinless
  chicken
2.5 cm/1 inch piece of fresh
  ginger, peeled and sliced
2 small garlic cloves, peeled
  and sliced
2 teaspoons cornflour
1 tablespoon soy sauce

1 tablespoon dry sherry
150 ml/¹/₄ pint chicken stock
1 tablespoon sunflower oil
50 g/2 oz unsalted shelled
  cashew nuts
salt and pepper
4 spring onions, finely sliced
  lengthways

Trim the chicken of all fat and cut into even-sized pieces. Put the pieces in a bowl with the ginger and garlic. Cover the bowl and leave to stand.

Mix the cornflour with the soy sauce, sherry and chicken stock.

Heat the oil in a wok or a large frying-pan. Add the cashew nuts and stir-fry until lightly browned. Remove with a slotted spoon and set aside.

Add the chicken with the ginger and garlic and stir-fry until the chicken is cooked and tender.

Add the liquid ingredients and stir until they are well blended and the liquid has thickened. Add a little water if it seems too thick.

Taste the sauce and season with salt and pepper if necessary.

Pile the chicken and sauce into a warmed serving dish and sprinkle the spring onions and cashew nuts on top.

FISH

Salmon steaks with tomato and basil

Serves 4

The pine kernels contain vitamin E and calcium.

4 175 g/6 oz salmon steaks
sunflower oil
10 tomatoes
1 onion, chopped
2 tablespoons chopped fresh
basil

salt and a little sugar
5 spring onions, chopped,
and 50 g/2 oz pine kernels
to garnish

Preheat the oven to Gas Mark 4/180 °C/350 °F.

Wipe the salmon steaks. Put each one on a fairly large, lightly oiled, round piece of tin foil.

Chop the tomatoes roughly. Put them in a large saucepan with the onion and 2 tablespoons of water. Cook the mixture very slowly until quite a lot of liquid seeps out of the tomatoes. Increase the heat and let the sauce simmer for 15 minutes.

Liquidize the sauce and push it through a sieve into a clean saucepan. Reduce it by rapid boiling to a thick consistency. Let it cool slightly and add the basil with a little sugar and salt to taste.

Divide the tomato mixture between the salmon steaks, wrap them up in the tin foil to form parcels and bake them in the oven for 15–20 minutes.

While the salmon steaks are cooking, stir-fry the pine kernels in a little sunflower oil. Be careful not to let them burn.

Just before serving, open the parcels slightly and sprinkle each one first with pine kernels and then with the spring onions.

Smoked salmon and dill filo tart

Serves 8

25 g/1 oz butter, melted
10–12 sheets filo pastry
175 g/6 oz smoked salmon
   trimmings
6 eggs

600 ml/1 pint low-fat fromage
   frais or extra thick half-fat
   cream
a few sprigs fresh dill
freshly ground black pepper

Lightly brush the base and sides of a 20 cm/8 inch deep loose-bottomed cake tin with melted butter. Line with layers of filo pastry brushed with butter, alternating the direction of each layer.

Preheat the oven to Gas Mark 3/170 °C/325 °F.

Place the salmon, eggs, fromage frais or cream, dill and pepper in a food processor and process for a few seconds.

Put the salmon mixture in the lined tin and bake in the oven for 40–50 minutes, or until just set.

Greek-style cod

Serves 4

4 cod steaks or filleted
  slices weighing about 1 kg/
  2 lb in total
6 tablespoons olive oil, plus
  extra for greasing
2 cloves garlic, sliced finely
4 tablespoons finely chopped
  fresh parsley

450 g/1 lb tomatoes, peeled,
  deseeded and finely
  chopped
2 tablespoons toasted
  breadcrumbs
salt and black pepper

Preheat the oven to Gas Mark 5/190 °C/375 °F.

Wash and dry the fish and arrange it in a medium-sized oiled baking dish.

Lightly beat together all the other ingredients, apart from the breadcrumbs. Spread some of this mixture over each slice of fish, sprinkle with breadcrumbs and bake for 30–40 minutes, basting occasionally, until light golden and crisp on top.

Serve with boiled new potatoes or brown rice and a green salad.

Fish pie

Serves 6

1.5 kg/3 lb potatoes, cubed
75 g/3 oz butter
salt and pepper
2 eggs
700 g/1½ lb smoked haddock
    fillet
2 bay-leaves
6 peppercorns
450 ml/¾ pint milk

1 leek, sliced thinly
50 g/2 oz plain flour
300 ml/½ pint white wine
3 tomatoes, skinned and
    quartered
50 g/2 oz Cheddar cheese,
    grated
1 tablespoon sesame seeds
salt and pepper to taste

Boil the potatoes until tender. Drain, add half the butter and some salt and pepper. Mash well and set aside.

Boil the eggs for 7 minutes, cool quickly in cold water and shell. Cut into quarters and set aside.

Place the haddock in a pan with the bay-leaves, peppercorns and milk. Bring to the boil, then cover and simmer for 12–15 minutes, until tender. Remove the fish, skin and flake into large pieces and set aside. Strain the milk.

Melt the remaining butter in a pan, add the leek and fry for 5 minutes, until softened. Stir in the flour and cook for 1 minute. Gradually stir in the reserved milk and wine and cook, stirring, until thickened. Remove from the heat and gently stir in the fish, tomatoes, eggs, salt and pepper.

Transfer to a 2.25 litre/4 pint ovenproof dish and cover with the mashed potato. Fork up the top of the pie and sprinkle with the cheese and sesame seeds. Cook in a preheated oven at Gas Mark 6/ 200 °C/400 °F for 20–25 minutes, until the top is golden brown. Serve hot.

Mackerel with lemon and onion

Serves 4

2 lemons
4 mackerel, each weighing
   225 g/8 oz, gutted and
   filleted
6 spring onions, chopped

a few dill sprigs
150 ml/¼ pint dry cider
2 bay-leaves
salt and pepper

Peel the lemons, discarding all pith, then slice the fruit thinly.

Arrange the lemon, spring onions and dill over one half of each fish and sprinkle with salt and pepper. Place the other fish half on top and secure with wooden cocktail sticks, if necessary.

Place in a greased baking dish, pour over the cider and add the bay-leaves. Cover with tin foil and cook in a preheated oven at Gas Mark 4/180 °C/350 °F for 30–40 minutes, until tender. Serve hot, with a side salad.

Herring salad

Serves 4

6 pickled herring fillets
1 red onion
1 apple
half a lettuce, shredded

DRESSING

150 ml/5 fl oz carton low-fat fromage frais
3 spring onions, chopped
1 tablespoon snipped chives
salt and pepper

Slice the herrings diagonally into strips. Cut the onion into quarters, then slice as thinly as possible. Quarter, core and slice the apple. Mix the herring, onion and apple together and set aside.

Mix together the fromage frais, spring onions, half the chives and some salt and pepper.

Arrange the lettuce on 4 individual plates. Top with the herring mixture and fromage frais dressing and sprinkle with the remaining chives.

Grilled trout with pesto and tomato sauce

Serves 4

2 tablespoons olive oil	4 trout, each weighing about
4 ripe tomatoes, skinned and	225 g/8 oz, gutted
chopped	2 tablespoons pesto
3 anchovy fillets, chopped	salt and pepper
finely (optional)	parsley sprigs to garnish

Heat the oil in a frying-pan, add the tomatoes and fry gently for about 5 minutes. Season with pepper and add the anchovies, if using. Keep warm.

Season the trout inside and out with salt and pepper. Cook under a preheated medium grill for 5–6 minutes on each side.

Just before serving, stir the pesto into the tomato sauce. Pour a little sauce over each fish and garnish with parsley sprigs to serve.

Smoked trout and watercress pâté

Serves 4–6

*1 smoked trout, weighing
    about 350 g/12 oz
1 bunch watercress
3 tablespoons freshly
    squeezed orange juice*

*100 g/4 oz curd cheese
50 g/2 oz butter, melted
salt and pepper
orange and cucumber slices to
    garnish*

Remove the skin and bones from the trout. Break the fish into several pieces, then place in a blender or food processor and process until fairly smooth.

Remove the tough stalks from the watercress. Put the leaves in the blender or processor with the fish until finely chopped. Transfer the mixture to a mixing bowl.

Stir in the remaining ingredients. Press into a small dish and smooth the top. Chill until required, then serve on individual plates, garnished with orange and cucumber slices.

Baked fish pasta

Serves 4

1 tablespoon vegetable oil
1 onion, chopped
1 carrot, chopped
1 celery stick, chopped
400 g/14 oz can tomatoes
150 ml/¼ pint vegetable stock
1 tablespoon pesto

175 g/6 oz wholemeal pasta
  shells
450 g/1 lb cod fillet, skinned
  and cubed
175 g/6 oz low-fat mozzarella
  cheese, sliced thinly
salt and pepper

Heat the oil in a saucepan, add the onion and fry until softened. Add the carrot and celery and cook for 5 minutes. Add the tomatoes with their juice, the stock, salt and pepper and bring to the boil. Simmer, uncovered, for 10–15 minutes, until thickened, then stir in the pesto. Remove from heat.

Meanwhile, cook the pasta according to packet instructions, drain and place in an oiled 1.75 litre/3 pint ovenproof dish.

Add the fish to the pasta and mix well. Pour over the sauce and mix lightly. Arrange the mozzarella cheese over the top. Cook in a preheated oven at Gas Mark 5/190 °C/375 °F for 25 minutes, until the cheese topping has melted. Serve with a green salad.

PASTA

Pasta with tomato and egg sauce

Serves 4

2 large onions, sliced
1 tablespoon olive oil
2 400 g/14 oz cans chopped
   tomatoes
300 g/10 oz wholemeal or
   spinach (green) pasta
   shapes

1 tablespoon chopped fresh
   basil
3 eggs, beaten lightly
fresh Parmesan cheese,
   grated
salt and pepper

Cook the onions very slowly in the olive oil for 15–20 minutes. They should become soft but not coloured.

Add the tomatoes, salt and pepper, stir well and bring the mixture to the boil. Simmer for 10 minutes.

Meanwhile, cook the pasta in rapidly boiling water to which a teaspoon of oil and a little salt has been added. When cooked, drain well and refresh with hot water.

Take the tomato sauce off the heat, season with salt and pepper, add the basil and then gradually pour in the lightly beaten eggs. The sauce should become rich and creamy.

Mix a little of the sauce with the pasta, pile it into a serving dish and pour the remaining sauce over it.

Serve sprinkled with a little freshly grated Parmesan cheese.

Wholemeal tagliatelli with peppers

Serves 4

Peppers are a good source of vitamin A.

1 red pepper
1 yellow pepper
2 cloves garlic, sliced
6 tablespoons olive oil
450 g/1 lb wholemeal
  tagliatelli

4 tablespoons grated
  Parmesan cheese
a small bunch fresh
  coriander, chopped finely
salt and freshly ground black
  pepper

Cut the peppers into quarters and grill them skin-side up until the skins blister and can be easily peeled off. Cut into strips.

Gently fry the garlic in 2 tablespoons of oil until soft, then stir in the peppers and cook for another minute or two. Season generously with salt and pepper and add the rest of the oil.

Boil the tagliatelli, drain and then toss in the pepper mixture. Stir in the grated cheese and the coriander, adjust the seasoning and serve at once.

Red lentil lasagne

Serves 4–6

2 teaspoons olive oil
1 large onion, chopped
1 clove garlic, crushed
1 red or green pepper,
  deseeded and chopped
100 g/4 oz mushrooms,
  thickly sliced
2 teaspoons chopped fresh
  basil

2 teaspoons chopped fresh
  oregano
225 g/8 oz red split lentils
400 g/14 oz can chopped
  tomatoes
1 bay-leaf
salt and pepper
100 g/4 oz wholemeal lasagne
  (about 8 sheets)

SAUCE

25 g/1 oz margarine
25 g/1 oz wholemeal flour
300 ml/½ pint skimmed milk
½ teaspoon mustard powder
75 g/3 oz low-fat Cheddar cheese, grated

Heat the oil in a large pan and gently fry the onion and garlic over a moderate heat for 5 minutes. Add the pepper and mushrooms and cook for 5 minutes. Add the basil, oregano and lentils and cook gently for 2–3 minutes. Stir in the tomatoes and their juice with 300 ml/½ pint of water and the bay-leaf.

Bring to the boil, cover, and simmer for 20–25 minutes, until the lentils are soft. Add a little extra water if the mixture seems too dry. Season with salt and pepper, then remove the bay-leaf.

Meanwhile, put the lasagne in a large saucepan of boiling water and simmer for 8–10 minutes, until just tender. Drain, put in a bowl and cover with cold water.

To make the sauce: melt the margarine in a small pan and stir in the flour. Stir it while it cooks over a gentle heat for 3–4 minutes. Remove from the heat and gradually stir in the milk. Bring to the boil, stirring all the time, until the sauce thickens. Cook gently for 3–4 minutes, still stirring constantly. Remove from the heat and beat in the mustard powder and most of the cheese. Check the seasoning.

Put a third of the lentil mixture into the base of a deep casserole or ovenproof dish. Cover with a third of the lasagne, then add another third of the lentils, followed by another third of the lasagne. Cover this with half the cheese sauce, then with the rest of the lentils. Top with the remaining lasagne. Pour the rest of the cheese sauce over the top and sprinkle with the cheese.

Bake in a preheated oven at Gas Mark 4/180 °C/350 °F for 30–35 minutes, until bubbling and golden brown. Serve hot.

Pasta in ginger and tomato sauce

Serves 4

2 teaspoons olive oil
1 onion, finely chopped
4 celery sticks, trimmed and
    finely chopped
2 tablespoons finely chopped
    fresh root ginger
700 g/1½ lb can peeled
    tomatoes
2 teaspoons chopped
    marjoram

3 tablespoons tomato purée
375 g/12 oz wholemeal
    macaroni
1 teaspoon lemon juice
salt and pepper
grated Parmesan cheese and
    chopped parsley to garnish

To make the sauce, first heat the oil in a medium-sized saucepan and gently fry the onion and celery for 5 minutes, until soft. Add the ginger and cook gently for a further 2 minutes to allow the flavours to blend.

Add the tomatoes, marjoram and tomato purée. Bring to the boil. Reduce the heat and simmer for 15 minutes, until the tomatoes are cooked.

Meanwhile, cook the macaroni by simmering in 2.5 litres/4 pints of water with a little lemon juice for 10 minutes.

When the macaroni is cooked, drain well. Mix with the sauce, season and serve garnished with Parmesan cheese and chopped parsley.

NUTS, SEEDS AND GRAINS

Sesame-crusted aubergines

Serves 4

2 small aubergines
2 teaspoons fine sea salt
2 tablespoons tahini (sesame
   paste)
2 tablespoons tomato purée
juice of 1 lemon

1 clove garlic, crushed
1 teaspoon paprika
dash of Tabasco sauce
2 tablespoons sesame or
   sunflower oil
4 tablespoons sesame seeds

Cut the aubergines in half lengthways, score the cut surfaces twice and sprinkle with the salt. Leave, cut side down, in a colander for 30 minutes to drain.

Put the tahini in a bowl and work in the tomato purée, lemon juice, garlic, paprika and Tabasco sauce to make a smooth paste.

Heat the grill to high. Rinse the aubergines under cold water and dry with paper towels. Brush with oil. Lay them on the grill rack, cut-side down, and grill for 2–3 minutes, until they begin to feel soft. Turn them over and cook for a further 2 minutes.

Spread the cut sides of the aubergine halves with the tahini paste and sprinkle the sesame seeds on top.

Return the aubergines to the grill for 1 minute to brown the sesame seeds.

Tahini dip

Serves 4

5 tablespoons tahini (sesame
   paste)
150 ml/¼ pint warm water
1–2 cloves garlic

6 tablespoons lemon juice
4 tablespoons vegetable oil
salt

Combine in a blender the tahini, water, garlic and salt and blend.
   Slowly add the lemon and oil, alternating them, while the blades
are in motion, until the mixture looks creamy in colour and texture.

Hazelnut salad

Serves 4

> 1 round lettuce heart
> 6 spring onions
> 225 g/8 oz white cherries
> 225 g/8 oz shelled hazelnuts

DRESSING

a further 25 g/1 oz shelled hazelnuts	*1 teaspoon Dijon mustard*
6 tablespoons buttermilk	*1 teaspoon clear honey*
4 tablespoons sherry vinegar	*sea salt*
	freshly ground pepper

Begin by toasting the hazelnuts for the dressing in a dry, heavy-based pan for 3 minutes. Place all the remaining dressing ingredients in a blender and blend to a smooth cream. Set aside to allow the flavours to develop and mingle.

Separate the lettuce leaves. Wash and drain well, then arrange on 4 individual serving plates.

Thinly slice the spring onions diagonally. Scatter over the lettuce, or arrange in an attractive mound in the centre of each plate.

Stone the cherries and decorate the plates with them.

Toast the remaining hazelnuts until evenly browned. Scatter over each plate. Serve at once, offering the dressing in a sauce-boat.

Seeded potato and corn cakes

Serves 4–6

225 g/8 oz potatoes, peeled,
  washed and grated
1 small onion, finely chopped
1 clove garlic, crushed
75 g/3 oz blanched sweetcorn
1 tablespoon chopped fresh
  parsley
2 large free-range eggs, beaten
1½ tablespoons wholemeal
  flour

1 tablespoon toasted
  sunflower seeds
1 tablespoon toasted flaked
  almonds
1 teaspoon cumin seeds
sea salt
freshly ground black pepper
vegetable oil for frying

In a large bowl, beat together all the ingredients except the oil to form a stiff batter.

Heat a little oil in a large frying pan and drop in heaped tablespoons of the mixture, 4 at a time, to sauté. They will spread to form little pancakes. When golden underneath, turn and sauté until cooked on the other side.

Serve hot or cold.

Almond paella

Serves 4

2 teaspoons sunflower oil
1 onion, chopped
1 clove garlic
75 g/3 oz whole almonds,
  blanched
175 g/6 oz long-grain brown
  rice
1 stick celery, chopped
225 g/8 oz green summer
  vegetables, such as leeks,
  broccoli or mangetout peas

1 small green pepper, sliced
1 teaspoon cumin seeds,
  crushed
2 teaspoons fresh marjoram
2 bay-leaves
1 teaspoon soy sauce or salt
  and pepper
1 tablespoon lemon juice

Heat the oil in a large pan and fry the onion and garlic for 5 minutes. Add the almonds and rice and cook for 5 minutes.

Add the chopped celery, green vegetables, green pepper, cumin seeds and marjoram. Cook gently for a further 5 minutes.

Stir in the bay-leaves and 600 ml/1 pint boiling water. Bring to the boil, cover and simmer for 30 minutes, until the rice is cooked and the liquid has been absorbed.

Add the soy sauce or salt and pepper, and the lemon juice. Remove the bay-leaves and serve hot.

Useful addresses

National Association for Premenstrual Syndrome (NAPS)
PO Box 72
Sevenoaks
Kent TN13 1QX
Tel. 01732 459378

The Premenstrual Society (PREMSOC)
PO Box 429
Addlestone
Surrey KT15 1DZ

The Women's Nutritional Advisory Service
PO Box 268
Lewes
East Sussex BN7 2QN
Tel. 01273 487366

Alcohol Concern
275 Gray's Inn Road
London WC1X 8QF
Tel. 0171 928 7377

MIND (National Society For Mental Health)
22 Harley Street
London W1N 2ED

QUIT (National Society of Non-Smokers)
102 Gloucester Place
London W1H 3DA
Tel. 0171 388 5775; Quitline 0800 002200

The Health Education Authority
Hamilton House
Mabledon Place
London WC1H 9TX
Tel. 0171 383 3833

Marie Stopes International
108 Whitfield Street
London W1P 6BE
Tel. London 0171 388 2585/388 0662/388 4843; Leeds 0113 244 0685; Manchester 0161 832 4260

Further reading

Evennett, Karen, *Coping Successfully with PMS*. Sheldon, 1995.
Evennett, Karen, *Women's Health: An Essential Guide for the Modern Woman*. Cassell, 1996.
Eyton, Audrey, *The F-Plan*. Penguin, 1982.
Stewart, Maryon and Abraham, Guy, *Beat PMS through Diet*. Vermilion, 1994.

Recipe books
Brown, Sarah, *Vegetarian Cookery*. Dorling Kindersley, 1988.
Cadogan, Mary, *Fish and Shellfish*. Woodhead-Faulkner and J. Sainsbury plc, 1987.
Conil, Jean and Franklin, Fay, *French Vegetarian Cooking*. Thorsons, 1987.
Duff, Gail, *Wholefood Cookery for Everyone*. Woodhead-Faulkner and J. Sainsbury plc, 1986.
Ellis, Audrey, *High Fibre Cookbook*. Hamlyn, 1985.
Grigson, Jane, *Cooking Carrots*. Abson Books, 1980.
Richardson, Rosamund, *The Vegetarian Gourmet*. Woodhead-Faulkner and J. Sainsbury plc, 1987.
Salaman, Rena, *The Cooking of Greece and Turkey*. Woodhead-Faulkner and J. Sainsbury plc, 1989.
Smith, Michael, *The Homes and Gardens Cook Book*. Allen Lane, 1982.
Waldegrave, Caroline, *The Low-Fat Gourmet*. Woodhead-Faulkner and J. Sainsbury plc, 1989.

Index